Primary and Emer

Primary and Emergency Dental Care

A Practitioner's Guide

Edited by

K. H. Figures
Director, School of Dental Hygiene, The Charles Clifford Dental Hospital, Sheffield

and

D. J. Lamb
Senior Lecturer/Honorary Consultant, Department of Restorative Dentistry, University of Sheffield

WRIGHT

Wright
An imprint of Butterworth-Heinemann Ltd
Linacre House, Jordan Hill, Oxford OX2 8DP

A member of the Reed Elsevier group

OXFORD LONDON BOSTON
MUNICH NEW DELHI SINGAPORE SYDNEY
TOKYO TORONTO WELLINGTON

First published 1995

British Library Cataloguing in Publication Data
A catalogue record of this book is available from the British Library.

ISBN 0 7326 1013 4

Library of Congress Cataloguing in Publication Data
A catalogue record for this book is available from the Library of Congress.

Typeset by Latimer Trend & Co Ltd, Plymouth
Printed and bound by Hartnolls Limited, Bodmin, Cornwall

Contents

List of contributors

A. C. Crosby FRCS(Edin)
Consultant in Accident and Emergency Medicine, Royal Hallamshire Hospital, Sheffield

Lesley E. Davidson MSc BDS FDSRCS(Edin) DOrthRCS(Eng)
Consultant in Paediatric Dentistry, The Charles Clifford Dental Hospital, Sheffield

K. H. Figures MDS BDS FDSRCS(Edin)
Director, School of Dental Hygiene, The Charles Clifford Dental Hospital, Sheffield

D. J. Lamb MDS BDS FDSRCS(Eng)
Senior Lecturer/Honorary Consultant, Department of Restorative Dentistry, University of Sheffield

Simon Northeast PhD BDS FDSRCS(Edin)
Department of Restorative Dentistry, University of Sheffield

P. S. Rothwell MDS DDS DGDP (UK)
Professor of Dental Services, Department of Dental Services, University of Sheffield

Nigel Thomas BDS MCDH DDPH RCS
Consultant in Dental Public Health, Rotherham and Doncaster

Trevor F. Walsh DDS MSc BDS FDS RCS(Eng)
Professor and Consultant in Restorative Dentistry, School of Clinical Dentistry, University of Sheffield

Philip Wragg BDS FDSRCS(Edin) DRDRCS(Edin)
Consultant in Restorative Dentistry, The Charles Clifford Dental Hospital, Sheffield

Preface

The treatment of emergencies is within the remit of the general dental practitioner but it is difficult to give broad clinical experience in coping with dental emergencies to undergraduates. In general practice, with the multitude of techniques available it is sometimes difficult for the experienced practitioner to know which approach would be best and the recently qualified practitioner can be particularly at a disadvantage. It was felt that a book was needed which would offer guidance on primary and emergency care techniques, but written mainly from a restorative perspective. The various contributors have considerable experience in their subject areas and also in coping with the emergencies which present. The final text we hope is informative and offers sensible advice for the delivery of primary and emergency care to patients who are dentally distressed.

KHF
DJL

1

The clinical environment

Trevor Walsh

Introduction

As if the range of clinical problems that general dental practitioners come across were not enough, before they even see their first patient dentists must be aware of a wide range of related matters. This chapter contains information on those aspects which are essential if clinicians are to practise legally and safely and maintain their equipment and their patients' rights. The subjects are:

- General Dental Council regulations
- Health & safety
- Medico-legal matters
- General anaesthesia, sedation and resuscitation
- Hospital and specialist referrals
- Control of cross-infection.

General Dental Council regulations

To engage in the practice of dentistry in the UK requires the practitioner to be registered in accordance with the Dentists Act 1984. To be on the Dentists Register evidence will be required of:

- identity
- good character
- requisite skill and knowledge; either a UK diploma or degree, or an approved recognized overseas diploma
- necessary knowledge of English
- good health, both physical and mental
- payment of the approved annual fee.

Registration will entitle the dentist to use the description of dentist, dental surgeon or dental practitioner and undertake the practice of dentistry. The latter is defined as 'the performance of any operation or treatment or attendance usually performed or given by dentists'. This includes any procedures connected with the fitting, insertion or fixing of dentures, artificial teeth or other dental appliances. The only exceptions to this prohibition are:

- registered dental or medical students
- registered dental auxiliaries
- registered medical practitioners.

In the near future in the UK, no dentist will be able to enter general dental practice as a principal without having undergone a structured period of vocational training. The basic dental degree or diploma is just the first stage in an educational experience that should last the lifetime of the dentist. In view of continuing changes in oral and dental diseases and in patterns of dental care, flexibility and determination to learn new procedures and techniques are essential if a dentist is to retain 'the requisite knowledge and skill for the efficient practice of dentistry'.

For those wishing to specialize in an aspect of dentistry, it is important to obtain wide general experience, including that in hospitals, before embarking on more specialized training. Thereafter all dentists should maintain and update their professional skills, for example by attendance at courses, clinical attachments in hospitals, and attendance at professional meetings.

Newly qualified dental graduates, after completing their period of vocational training, will usually look for associate positions in existing practices. A careful inspection of the surgery where one hopes to be employed is usually the start of the decision process. The following should be taken into account when choosing an associate position:

- Will you have your own surgery? Will it be shared or will you have to work in more than one surgery? It is obviously preferable to have a stable base from which to work.
- Check the equipment. Does it work efficiently? Check the following items:
  - Unit and chair
  - Aspiration, which preferably should be centrally ducted
  - Handpieces: they should be sufficient in number to sterilize between patients, and a straight handpiece should also be provided. Check that there is a good range of conventional and air turbine burs. If there is not, get a commitment from the principal or practice manager that these will be provided

Ultrasonic or sonic scaler
Autoclave
Amalgamator
Light curing unit
X-ray unit.

- Ask how the instruments are delivered. A tray system is desirable.
- Ask to see the endodontic kit. This should include files, Gates–Glidden drills, paper and GP points, as well as a rubber dam kit.
- Check on control of infection procedures. Protective spectacles should be provided for you and your dental nurse. A 'sharps box' must be provided, and the practice should have explicit protocols for the disposal of waste. There should be two sinks with hot and cold water, as well as disinfectant detergents for hand washing.
- Finally check on the general condition of the surgery. Is it light and airy, with adequate ventilation and heating? There should be vinyl flooring in the clinical area as well as storage units, and it should have adequate work surfaces.

Remember that you may be obliged to work out the term of any agreed contract, so it is important that you are satisfied with the working conditions.

Health and safety

Although this book is concerned with the problems and complications in restorative dental practice, attention to health and safety will help to prevent many problems and allow effective action to be taken when an unforeseen event does occur. However, the advice given in this chapter does not aim to cover comprehensively all aspects of health and safety in restorative dentistry. For that the reader is referred to the excellent guide produced by the British Dental Association (*Health and safety law for dental practices*).

The dentist's responsibilities for health and safety are governed by the Health and Safety at Work, etc. Act (1974). This seeks to protect all persons at work, including the general public, who may be affected by work activities. We have a general duty as employers under the Act to ensure, as far as is reasonably practicable, the health, safety and welfare at work of our staff, our patients and ourselves.

In general a dentist's responsibilities as an employer are:

- to make his or her practice safe and without risks to health

- to keep dust, fumes and noise under control
- to ensure equipment is safe and that safe systems of work are identified and followed
- to ensure that articles and substances are moved, stored and used safely
- to provide adequate welfare facilities
- to give information, instruction, training and supervision necessary for health and safety.

Even associates or the self-employed have legal duties, which include:

- taking reasonable care of your own health and safety, and that of others who may be affected by what you do, or do not do
- co-operating with your employer on health and safety
- not interfering with or misusing anything provided for your health, safety or welfare.

The following are required by law:

A safety policy

All practices should display an official health and safety poster or provide each employee with a written policy. For practices with five or more employees this is mandatory. An approved poster entitled 'Health and safety law – what you should know' (ISBN 0-11-701424-9) is available. A suggested format for a dental practice advice policy is shown in the BDA advice sheet A3.

Fire precautions

Written fire procedure notices should be displayed and brought to the attention of all employees. Anyone working in the practice should know:

- where the nearest fire alarm is
- where the nearest fire appliance is
- how to use the fire appliances
- the fire escape route
- the fire assembly point.

Under the Fire Precautions Act 1971 a fire certificate may be required. The local fire protection officer will be able to give advice. Fire hazards should be minimized by ensuring that passages, hallways and exits are unobstructed. Flammable substances should be identified and stored safely. The procedures to be followed after the outbreak of fire should be understood by all staff, and this should include provisions for dealing with patients or visitors.

Premises

The premises must be kept in a safe condition, without risks to health. In addition to the Health and Safety at Work Act, dentists' premises are covered by the Occupiers' Liability Act 1957.

The following should be considered:

- Entrances and exits should be safe.
- Passages, stairs and gangways should not be obstructed.
- Stairs and steps should be well lit, with firm, secure handrails.
- Floors should have non-slip surfaces and floor coverings should be secure.
- Ceilings and walls should be washable and free from dust traps.
- Furnishing and fittings should be without sharp edges.
- Fires and heaters should be guarded and be without trailing leads. They should be out of reach of children.

Visual Display Units

The Health and Safety (Display Screen Equipment) Regulations 1992 came into force in 1993 and cover the design and use of computer workstations. New equipment will be constructed to comply with the regulations, but existing equipment will need to comply by 1997. Staff who regularly use VDU equipment will be entitled to eyesight tests and appropriate corrective appliances.

Welfare arrangements

The Workplace (Health, Safety and Welfare) Regulations 1992 cover four broad areas:

- the working environment
- safety
- facilities
- housekeeping.

Dental practices should comply with the following:

Working environment

The workplace should normally be at a temperature of at least 16°C, and allow work without the need for special clothing. Lighting should be sufficient to enable staff to work safely and without experiencing eye strain. If windows do not provide sufficient ventilation, mechanical ventilation systems should be provided as appropriate. Rooms should be sufficiently large to enable staff and visitors to move around with ease. As a guide, the total volume of the room, when empty, divided by the number of people working in it should be at least 11 m^3. Workstations should be arranged so that tasks can be carried out safely and comfortably. The seating should support the lower back and be appropriate for the task.

Safety

Floor surfaces should be even, free from holes, and have a non-slip surface so as not to cause a person to trip, slip or fall, or to drop anything being carried. Windows and skylights should be constructed to enable them to be opened, closed and cleaned safely from the inside. Doors and gates should have a transparent panel unless they are low enough to be seen over. Glazed doors and partitions should be made of a safety material or be protected against breakage, for example by obvious marking.

Facilities

Toilets and washing facilities should be sufficient for the number of employees and accessible. A changing room should be provided for workers who need to work in special clothing. Drying facilities must be provided if necessary. Effective measures should be taken to provide secure storage of clothing and personal belongings. Rest areas where staff can relax and eat their meals at work should be provided. 'No smoking' areas should be made available, but there is no requirement for smoking areas.

Housekeeping

The workplace and equipment should be maintained in efficient working order and good repair. Records should be kept to demonstrate that this requirement has been complied with. The standard of cleanliness required depends on the use of the workplace: a surgery would therefore be expected to have a high level of cleanliness, which should include floors, walls and ceilings.

First Aid

Under the Health and Safety (First-Aid) Regulations 1981 all workplaces must have first-aid provision, appropriate to the degree of hazard associated with the workplace and the number of people employed.

The relatively small number of people who usually work in a practice means that there is no legal requirement for dentists to provide a first-aider; but it is advisable to do so. If a competent first-aider is not available, an employer must ensure that, at all times when people are at work, a person has been appointed to take charge of any medical emergency (for example to call an ambulance) in the event of serious illness or injury. All dental practices must have a first-aid box containing only items that a first-aider or appointed person has been trained to use. They should not contain medication of any kind. The Health and Safety Executive recommend that first-aid boxes should contain the following items:

- a guidance card
- 20 individually wrapped sterile adhesive dressings (assorted sizes)
- 2 sterile eye pads
- 6 individually wrapped triangular bandages
- 6 safety pins
- 6 medium-sized individually wrapped sterile unmedicated wound dressings (approximately 13 cm × 9 cm)
- 3 extra large sterile individually wrapped unmedicated wound dressings (approximately 28 cm × 17.5 cm)
- 10 individually wrapped moist clean wipes.

Sterile water or sterile normal saline in sealed disposable containers should be provided where tap water is not available for eye irrigation. Each container should hold at least 300 ml of solution.

Accident notification and reporting

The Reporting of Injuries, Diseases and Dangerous Occurrences Regulations came into force in 1986. These cover all persons at work, including the self-employed and members of the public. There is an important provision to exclude accidents to patients when they are undergoing treatment in a hospital or the surgery of a doctor or dentist. The Health and Safety Executive must be notified of any accident causing death or major injury, and of any dangerous occurrence. These must be reported promptly, by telephone if possible, with written confirmation on Form F2508 (available from HMSO, ISBN 0-11-883853-9).

Hazards in the Dental Surgery

There are a large number of hazards in the dental surgery, and the main ones are associated with:

- infection risks
- anaesthetics gases
- toxic substances
- lasers
- electricity
- medicines
- mercury
- ionizing radiation
- water supplies.

Infection risks

These may be posed by aerosols, cross-infection and pathology specimens. Aerosols may contain oil, tooth particles, bacteria, fungi and possibly viruses, and may be generated by air turbines, ultrasonic scalers or triple syringes. Risks of infection may be reduced by good ventilation and the use of high-speed aspiration, face masks and protective spectacles. The use of a chlorhexidine mouth rinse prior to using high-speed equipment will also reduce the microbial burden of aerosols.

We all have a duty to protect our patients and staff from the risk of cross-infection. A practical routine for the prevention of infection and cross-infection should be followed with every patient treated. The reader is referred to the BDA's advice sheet *The control of cross-infection*. It is also essential that equipment sent to laboratories for repair should be sterilized or adequately decontaminated before dispatch.

Protective clothing can also minimize cross-infection, although it is not a substitute for more basic safety measures. Gloves should be worn for all clinical procedures, and should be replaced when damaged, since this will minimize contact with blood, serum and saliva. Eye protection should be worn by all dental personnel working near the patient during treatment. Spectacles should have full lenses and side protection, as half lenses do not give enough protection against splatter. Good-quality face masks give some protection against aerosol, but more importantly, give protection against splatter.

Clinical clothing should be worn only in surgery or laboratory and not taken into eating areas or the home. Contaminated clinical clothing should be washed on the hot wash cycle at a minimum temperature of 80°C. Shoes should be solid, to protect against mercury, pathogens and toxic substances.

Biopsy specimens sent to pathology laboratories for diagnostic opinions or tests must comply with packaging requirements issued by the Post Office. Only first class letter post or data post services may be used, and the parcel post service must not be used for specimens. These must be enclosed in a primary container of a capacity not exceeding 50 ml, hermetically sealed and wrapped in absorbent material to soak up any leakage in the event of damage, with the whole sealed in an outer leak-proof plastic bag. The Post Office recommend the use of a padded bag as an additional outer cover. The outer wrapping must be conspicuously labelled 'PATHOLOGICAL SPECIMEN FRAGILE WITH CARE'. It must show the name and address of the sender who is to be contacted in case of damage or leakage.

Dentists are responsible for sorting their waste, storing it safely and securely in a suitable container, and arranging for its safe disposal. Wastes should be divided into clinical and non-clinical items. Clinical waste should be stored in yellow containers and disposed of by high-temperature incineration. Sharps such as needles and scalpel blades must be sealed in a rigid puncture-proof 'sharps' container (to BS 7320) before disposal. Arrangements for clinical waste should be made with either a private contractor, a local authority or Family Health Services Authorities. Non-clinical waste should be stored in suitable containers or sacks, which should be securely tied and not overfilled. For most dental practices the local authority will collect non-clinical waste.

Anaesthetic gases

It has been suggested that prolonged exposure to anaesthetic gases may increase the risk of abortion or birth abnormalities. This may be minimized if equipment is well maintained and used with an effective scavenging system in a surgery that is well ventilated.

Toxic substances

As many of the substances used in a dental practice are hazardous, toxic or allergenic in some way, the Control of Substances Hazardous to Health (COSHH) Regulations 1988, apply. The general aim of the Regulations is to make employers aware of the hazards at work and to encourage them to make the working environment safer. Employers must assess the risk to employees of all hazardous substances and decide on the action needed to remove or reduce these risks, and then implement appropriate action. Toxic substances can harm the body through inhalation, ingestion or contact with skin or eyes. An important key to the reduction of risk is the training of staff. Toxic substances used in surgeries include chemical disinfectants, such as alcohol, alcohol mixtures, hypochlorite disinfectants and aldehydes (e.g. formaldehyde and glutaraldehyde) and methyl methacrylate and mercury.

Lasers

Lasers should conform to BS 7192, and laser equipment is classified from 1 to 4 depending on the power output. Users of class 3B or 4 lasers are required to register with the District Health Authority under the Nursing Homes Act 1975 (Nursing Homes (Laser) Regulations 1984). Warning signs must be displayed at every entrance to an area containing lasers, they should only be used by trained staff, and the patient must have given informed consent to laser treatment. All equipment should be regularly maintained according to the manufacturer's instructions.

Electrical hazards

The dentist's responsibilities concerning the supply and use of electricity are governed by the Electricity at Work Regulations 1989. The supply to all appliances must be correctly wired and fused and should be installed by registered contractors. Electrical equipment must also be checked and tested by an appropriately qualified person, usually an electrician, and records of this testing must be kept. A guidance note PM32 is available from HMSO booksellers (ISBN 0-11-885590-5).

Medicines

Medicines may deteriorate if stored in extremes of temperatures, damp, or direct sunlight and this may have serious clinical implications. Medicines should always be stored according to the manufacturer's recommendations. Emergency drugs should be kept securely but be accessible at all times; but it is advisable to keep all medicines in a locked cupboard. Regular stock checks should be carried out and surplus and outdated stocks destroyed, keeping amounts to the minimum required. Careful records of medicines should be kept.

Mercury hazards

Chronic mercury poisoning has a variety of symptoms, including headache, lassitude, anorexia, dyspepsia, pallor, personality changes, tremors and gingivitis. The dangers of mercury poisoning may be reduced by attention to:

- training of personnel in the hazards of mercury
- personal hygiene measures
- careful clinical use
- a safe working environment, including effective ventilation
- safe storage
- safe disposal of waste
- appropriate protocols for dealing with spillage.

The use of mercury should be confined to areas that have impervious surfaces and are suitably lipped to facilitate the recovery of spilt mercury. Gloves should always be used. Particular care should be taken in the storage of mercury, as the use of inappropriate containers can lead to extensive contamination. A capsule system should preferably be used when restoring teeth with dental amalgam.

Radiation hazards

Dental radiography is covered by the Ionising Radiations Regulations 1985 and the Ionising Radiation (Protection of Persons Undergoing Medical Examination or Treatment) Regulations 1988, and these impose a number of statutory duties in relation to dental radiography and radiation protection, over and above the dentist's ethical and clinical responsibilities. To comply with the Acts, the practitioner must notify the Health and Safety Executive of the use of radiation in the practice and decide whether or not there is a need to appoint a Radiation Protection Adviser (RPA). All equipment should meet the standards recommended by the Standing Dental Advisory Committee (SDAC): a radiation safety assessment should be carried out every three years by a competent authority such as the National Radiological Protection Board, or the local or regional medical physics department. Appropriate education and training for all staff are required.

Dentists who delegate the task of taking dental radiographs must be satisfied that the person who takes the radiographs has received adequate training in conformity with the Regulations. DSAs should not take radiographs unless they are adequately trained and possess the core of knowledge required. Recognized courses are now available to provide DSAs with adequate training. Monitoring for staff is required if their individual workload exceeds 150 intra-oral or 50 panoral films per week.

Water supplies

Most water authorities require the isolation from the main supply of water used in dental equipment, such as that in hand-pieces, ultrasonic scalers, spittoons and triple syringes. This eliminates the possibility of back siphonage of contaminated water from the surgery to the main supply.

Medico-legal matters

An unavoidable aspect of current attitudes is the increasing intrusion of the law into all aspects of life, especially medicine and dentistry. The general public is less likely to accept that failed treatment is an act of God and is more likely to demand compensation from the practitioner involved. Not only does this make obtaining informed consent and dealing with complaints more important, but the general dental practitioner is more likely to be asked to prepare a legal report or to appear in court as an expert witness.

Consent

Dentists must obtain valid consent prior to carrying out treatment. For consent to be valid the dentist must himself or herself have explained to the patient the treatment proposed, the risks involved in the treatment, and alternative treatments. If an anaesthetic or sedation is to be given, all the procedures to be undertaken must be explained to the patient. The onus is on the dentist to ensure that all necessary explanations have been given to the patient, either by the dentist or by the anaesthetist. If a general anaesthetic or sedation is to be administered, consent must be obtained in writing.

The Department of Health has defined consent as 'the voluntary and continuing permission of the patient to receive a particular treatment. It must be based on adequate knowledge of the purpose, nature, likely effects and risks of that treatment including the likelihood of its success and any alternative to it.'. Thus, not only must the relevant facts be explained to the patient, but the practitioner must ensure that they are understood. How much advice is to be given and how consent should be recorded depends on the individual case. When a patient sits in the dental chair, it can be assumed that consent has been given for a non-invasive examination. Any invasive investigation, which may include radiographs, blood tests or periodontal probing, requires consent. Such consent would normally be obtained verbally, after the need for the investigation and possible consequences have been explained. Once the investigations are complete, the patient is entitled to advice on diagnosis and treatment planning, including possible treatment options or alternatives.

Patients cannot properly consider treatment options if they are not given information on sequelae and prognosis; but when the likely incidence of a possible complication is very slight, it is often considered in the best interests of patients not to warn them and thus risk frightening them unnecessarily. If there is an appreciable risk then a specific entry naming the complication should be made on the record card. Many claims involving paraesthesia or the need for immediate dentures are successful because it cannot be shown that the patient was specifically warned of possible post-operative complications. However, it is important to be aware that a pre-operative warning does not preclude a subsequent claim for negligence if the patient is dissatisfied with the standard of care received.

Cost is another important factor in consent. Without the knowledge of the financial implications of treatment, a patient cannot give a proper consent. Where treatment is to be protracted, involved or expensive, it is worthwhile writing to the patient with an explanation of the treatment, the time it will take, prognosis, sequelae and costs.

Language is an important element in obtaining consent. If the patient speaks a different language from the dentist, an interpreter may be required. Explanations should be simple and clear. The patient's failure to grasp information will be the dentist's responsibility, if it can be shown that the language of the explanation was not understood by the patient. Special care should be taken with deaf, partially sighted or blind patients.

Where treatment is unusual or experimental, patients must fully understand the proposed treatment, and it is worthwhile getting patients to sign statements to the effect that they accept the contentious nature of the therapy proposed.

In addition to communication difficulties, the dentist must consider the competence or ability of the patient to comprehend. Most children eventually reach an age where they can grasp relevant facts about their bodies. In the United Kingdom legislation permits an individual of sixteen years or over, and of sound mind, to give consent to dental treatment. Although the legislation does not preclude children under this age from giving consent, it is preferable to obtain this from both the child and the parent or guardian. If a parent or guardian is not available when children under sixteen years of age are examined, then extreme caution is advised. With an uncooperative child, there can be no justification for intimidation or for the use of physical force. In the case of an uncontrollable child, it may be better to cease treatment, make an appropriate explanation to the parent and arrange for necessary future treatment for the child. Consideration should be given to refusing treatment, except in an emergency, if concern remains about the understanding and agreement of both child and parent. Specific legislation, for example, the Children Act 1989 in the UK, defines parental responsibility and the consequent right to give consent to a child's treatment. Difficulties can arise; and, again, consideration should be given to the merit of withholding treatment if any doubt exists.

To be sure that consent has been obtained, an explanation of the investigations, their significance, the diagnosis, management options, sequelae, prognosis and costs should be given in sufficient detail to allow the patient, or person with parental responsibility, to understand the implications of treatment. The explanations must be given in a manner that the patient can fully understand. Only then will the patient be in a position to give consent. With minors, the dentist must also ensure that the person being given the information is the appropriate individual to give the consent.

Advertising and publicity

Dentists have a requirement only to use publicity or advertising material which is 'legal, decent and truthful' and has regard for professional propriety. All advertisements and advertising material relating to a given practice should include the name of at least one dentist normally in attendance at the practice. The material should not:

- be of a character that could reasonably be regarded as likely to bring the profession into disrepute;
- contain any reference to the efficiency, skills or knowledge of any other dentist or practice;
- make a claim which suggests superiority over any other dentist or practice; or
- recommend a specific product.

Publicity about dentists or their practices which arises through or from interviews with the media and which may bring the profession into disrepute should be avoided. The General Dental Council takes the view that those whose comments are invited by the media have a particular responsibility to ensure that their statements are factually accurate. It is important to distinguish between personal opinion or political belief and established facts. Whenever possible, you should request to see a proof of any article or statement before publication. In general the General Dental Council considers that any public statement which is calculated to mislead the public or damage public confidence in the profession constitutes serious professional misconduct.

Any advertisement, display or other information provided to the public should not include unrealistic descriptions of services offered at a practice. The name of every dentist regularly attending patients at a practice should be shown by means of a professional plate. In accordance with Section 26 of the Dentists Act, 1984, dentists may use in connection with their practices only those qualifications which are entered against their names in the Dentists Register and the title 'dentist', 'dental practitioner' or 'dental surgeon'. The letters 'Hons' with reference to an honours degree are not registrable, and may not, therefore, be used in connection with a dentist's practice. It also follows from this that dentists in the United Kingdom may not use the title 'Dr' in connection with their practices unless they are registered medical practitioners or possess doctorates which are entered against their names in the Dentists Register. However, all qualifications which dentists possess, whether registered or not, may appear in connection with their names in books on scientific or professional subjects, or articles or correspondence in professional journals. The names of persons other than dentists employed in the practice, such as dental hygienists, may not appear in advertisements or on signs outside the premises. No publicity or advertising material should indicate that a dentist has specialist expertise; but it may indicate that a practice is wholly or mainly devoted to particular types of treatment: for example, 'Practice limited to Periodontics'.

If advertising material includes reference to fees for professional advice or treatment, it should indicate:

- if items will be provided under the National Health Service regulations;
- whether any stated fee relates to treatment provided under the National Health Service regulations or under private contract;
- whether the stated fee is liable to vary; and
- that further details may be obtained on request.

Preparing dental reports

Many dental surgeons, although quite familiar with history taking, will feel uneasy about the prospect of preparing dental or legal reports. The request may be for an opinion on the clinical notes and other information (e.g. radiographs) or on the patient in person. The former is more likely where the solicitor is unsure whether to take the complaint further. When a full report is required the solicitor will ask for a factual account of the patient's present condition, the treatment provided by the practitioner against whom a complaint has been made, and an opinion on the appropriateness of the treatment. The test of whether treatment provided is negligent or not is 'the standard of the ordinary skilled man exercising and professing to have that special skill'. This means that the dentist must reach the standards expected of an ordinary skilled general practitioner, unless he or she is claiming to have additional skills such as an expertise in crown and bridgework or occlusal therapy.

To prevent misunderstandings afterwards, the practitioner should cost the time and materials involved in producing the report and obtain the solicitor's agreement in writing before seeing the patient or the clinical notes. The report should contain the following parts:

- full name and address of patient
- statement by the patient on [date]
- present complaints
- relevant medical history
- examination findings
- opinion on the findings
- signature and date.

The report should be sent with study models and copies of the radiographs to the solicitor. A covering letter should refer to any enclosures including models, radiographs, photographs and charts, as well as requesting the payment of any agreed fee. If the latter is different from the original quotation, then the reasons for the discrepancy should be stated.

Statement by the patient on [date]

This will usually be provided by the solicitor requesting the expert report. It should outline the history of the problem as stated by the patient.

Present complaints

If the complaints are lengthy it may be preferable to list them. It should be remembered that symptoms may be exaggerated and patients will try to put their best case forward. This may not be in their best interests, particularly if exaggeration can subsequently be proved; hence any discrepancies must be explored by the dentist providing the report. Any discrepancies or exaggeration may be commented on in the opinion section of the report.

Relevant medical history

Negative findings are important to demonstrate that the report has been thorough. Where there is a finding relevant to the complaint, this must be described.

Examination findings

This should constitute the major part of the report, and should include full clinical and radiographic findings. Copies of the radiographs should be provided with the report. In many cases the report may also include study casts and printed clinical photographs. This may be very important where the patient is having unsatisfactory work replaced by another practitioner.

Opinion on the findings

This section should be the only place in the dental report where the writer gives his opinion upon the previously stated facts. It is often useful to give an opinion on the statement of the patient and the state of the mouth as revealed by your examination. The report is frequently referring to the work of a colleague with the benefit of hindsight. Care should therefore be taken before condemning another practitioner's work. It is not always possible to produce excellent work, and the reporting practitioner cannot know the circumstances under which the work was undertaken. Consideration must be given to whether a reasonably competent practitioner would produce this standard of work. Often the nature of the work performed is understandable, but there has been no apparent explanation to the patient concerning the residual problems – for example when it has not been possible to fill a root canal completely. In these situations it is best to comment that 'the patient states that he/she was not informed of . . .'. If the opinion section of the report is lengthy then it may be appropriate to list your conclusions. The report should be signed and dated, and your qualifications should be shown.

Attending court as an expert witness

Concern has been expressed that many expert witnesses misunderstand their role in court. They should attend to give factual evidence, and not act as an advocate for one side or the other. Time spent in preparing for the case is well spent. The case notes should be revised, and a clear chronology of the events should be established. The expert witness would be well advised to attend court well before the time allotted to hearing the case to get the feel of the situation. Picking up any available information concerning the judge and his or her reputation and peculiarities would also be useful. It is important always to bear in mind that the function of the expert witness is to help the judge understand the case. Lawyers often complain that they cannot understand medical evidence. Witnesses should avoid being didactic, bombastic, self-important or self-opinionated. They should also remember that any written opinion will have been disclosed to the opposing legal representatives before the case is heard in court.

The following excellent advice has been given for the expert witness (Wake 1993):

- Expert evidence given in court should be independent and uninfluenced by the personalities involved in the litigation.
- An unbiased opinion should be given. The expert witness should not assume the role of an advocate.
- It should be made clear when a question or issue falls outside the witness's expertise.
- All facts or assumptions upon the opinion should be stated, together with any facts which may detract from the conclusions.
- If an opinion has few supporting data this must be admitted.
- If the expert comes to doubt his conclusions on a matter, then this must be communicated to the legal representatives without delay. The other side will then be informed.

Occasionally, the expert will not be asked to give evidence, but to be present in court to feed questions to the barrister to put to the opposition experts in order to discredit their evidence. It should also be remembered that very few cases actually come to trial, and most are settled before the hearing. The early availability of sensible, open advice from an expert may prevent many complaints ever reaching court. The even earlier provision of explanations to dissatisfied patients of why something has occurred may stop them seeking legal advice in the first place. (This is discussed in the next section.)

Complaints

The number of complaints about dental treatment has been steadily increasing. Several factors have encouraged patients to complain:

- the greater expectations raised by the Patient's Charter
- greater awareness of rights as consumers of a service
- a demand for greater accountability from the profession
- increased expectations as patients have opted for private treatment
- a tendency to wish to blame someone when things go wrong.

The NHS time limits for making a complaint are currently 13 weeks from the time of the incident. In most cases patients simply want to know what has happened or to receive an apology for some perceived injustice. When they seek an explanation or an apology they must be treated with courtesy and heard by the dentist in private surroundings with a sympathetic approach. Remedial treatment should be provided when this is possible, and this may prevent the case from going further. Dentists who tell patients to 'get lost' are only inviting trouble for themselves. A conciliatory initial approach is most important in avoiding a lengthy formal investigation by a third party. Hence dental practitioners must develop a practice-based informal complaints procedure. A written explanation should be sent to the patient within one week. If patients, after this conciliation, indicate that they will be taking their complaints further, practitioners would be well advised to inform their protection society.

In deciding whether to defend an action, the practitioner should bear in mind that the following criteria will be taken into account by the protection society:

- Is there a clear and complete statement from the defendant concerning the claim?
- Are there accurate, legible and contemporaneous written records and a complete set of radiographs and study casts, if these are appropriate?
- Is the defendant prepared to go to court?
- Does the defendant have a bearing and demeanour which would encourage support in court?
- Will the defendant perform competently in the witness box against possible hostile questioning?

- Is there a supportive expert witness for the defendant?
- Is there a figure to be settled which would make the risks and costs of defence at trial realistic?

All these factors must be considered before defending an action. The justice of the dentist's case is the least of the considerations in the decision to defend an action. Discovering the accusatorial system of British justice comes as a rude awakening to many in the dental profession.

Working with auxiliaries

Under Section 38 of the Dentists Act, 1984, it is unlawful for anyone to give, or even to suggest that they are prepared to give, any treatment or advice (including any treatment or advice in connection with the fitting, insertion or fixing of dentures, artificial teeth or other dental appliances) such as is normally given by a dentist, unless that person is registered in the Dentists Register or the Medical Register, or is an enrolled dental hygienist or dental therapist practising dentistry to the limited extent permitted by the Dental Auxiliaries Regulations, 1986 (as amended by the Dental Auxiliaries (Amendment) Regulations, 1991). This offence is termed covering.

Dentists who employ any person to practise dentistry have a duty to satisfy themselves that the person is permitted by law to practise, by inspecting their practising certificate or checking their registration status with the General Dental Council. A dentist who knowingly, or through neglect of this duty, enables a person to do dental work which that person is not permitted by law to do, is liable to proceedings for misconduct. Dentists would, therefore, be well advised to check annually the practising certificates of those they employ.

Dentists who employ dental auxiliaries should ensure that they are familiar with the work that those dental auxiliaries are entitled to carry out. Dentists should be aware that, where they practise in premises that are not self-contained but are shared with a dental laboratory, they could be held responsible for any illegal practice by the dental technicians working in the laboratory.

Dentists should not delegate responsibility for instructing patients in oral hygiene unless:

- they are satisfied that the person to whom the responsibility is delegated is fully competent to discharge it; and
- they understand that they are personally responsible for whatever instruction is given in their name.

A dentist who permits a dental hygienist to administer local infiltration analgesia or to work unsupervised must be satisfied that the dental hygienist is competent to do so. In order to be competent to administer local infiltration analgesia a dental hygienist must either:

- have completed additional training in local infiltration analgesia and gained a certificate in the administration of local infiltration analgesia; or
- have gained the Diploma (formerly Certificate of Proficiency) in Dental Hygiene more than twelve months after the coming into force of the Dental Auxiliaries (Amendment) Regulations, 1991; or
- hold the Certificate of Proficiency as a Dental Therapist in addition to the Diploma (formerly Certificate of Proficiency) in Dental Hygiene.

General anaesthesia, sedation and resuscitation

General anaesthesia is a risky procedure which should be avoided in dental practice if at all possible. Patients seeking general anaesthesia when it is not clinically appropriate should be persuaded to accept alternative techniques. Prior to the provision of general anaesthesia or sedation, careful consideration must be given to the need for the general anaesthesia, careful patient selection, and the skill and experience of the dentist, the anaesthetist and their team. In addition the dentist should consider the need for adequate facilities to monitor the patient, the use of complete and contemporaneous notes and adequate facilities for resuscitation.

When a general anaesthetic is administered it must be by a person, other than the dentist treating the patient, who must remain with the patient throughout the anaesthetic procedure, until the patient's protective reflexes have returned and the patient has recovered control of his or her own airway. This second person must be a dental or medical practitioner with appropriate postgraduate training and relevant experience in the use of anaesthetic drugs for dental purposes. The anaesthetist should be supported by an assistant specifically trained and experienced at assisting the monitoring of the patient's condition or in any emergency.

Careful clinical monitoring should be supplemented by the use of continuously-acting monitoring devices, and a defibrillator must be available. The dentist should also have the assistance of an appropriately trained dental surgery assistant. Formal training can be undertaken by the assistant to obtain the Certificate in Conscious Sedation of the National Examining Board for Dental Nurses. Where intravenous or inhalation sedation techniques are employed a suitably experienced practitioner may assume the responsibility of sedating the patient, as well as operating, provided that in the case of intravenous sedation the practitioner has undertaken relevant postgraduate training. As a minimum requirement a second appropriate person must be present throughout. Such an appropriate person might be a suitably trained dental nurse or dental auxiliary, whose experience and training enables him or her to monitor the patient. Should an emergency arise this person must also be capable of assisting the dentist. Suitable training for such persons would be provided by the Post-Certification Course for 'Assisting in the Care of the Patient relating to Treatment under Conscious Sedation', which has been drawn up by the Dental Surgery Assistants Standards and Training Advisory Board, or an equivalent.

When using sedation, the technique chosen should be the simplest that will enable successful treatment to be given, and in the case of intravenous sedation this will normally be by the use of a single drug. Where it is planned to use more than one drug for intravenous sedation continuously-acting monitoring devices must be used and a defibrillator must be available. The use of intravenous sedation for young children should be avoided. Where general anaesthesia or sedation is to be administered, a full medical history of the patient must be taken and patients must be given in advance clear and comprehensive pre- and post-treatment instructions in writing. Careful records of treatment and the procedure undertaken must be kept.

Neither general anaesthesia nor sedation should be employed unless proper equipment for their administration is used and adequate facilities, including appropriate drugs, for the resuscitation of the patient are readily available, with both the dentist and the staff fully trained in resuscitation techniques. Dentists must ensure that all those assisting them know precisely what is required of them should an emergency arise, and that they regularly practise their routine in a simulated emergency against the clock. It is essential that the equipment necessary for basic life support, including suction apparatus to clear the airway, oral airways to maintain it and positive-pressure equipment with appropriate attachments to inflate the lungs with oxygen, must already be set up and ready for use in the operating room. It is worth noting that equipment necessary for basic life support should be available in all dental practices.

Complete and adequate records of both the anaesthetic and the dental procedure are essential. A separate anaesthetic chart is preferable. The information on this should include:

- identification of the patient
- identification of the anaesthetist
- identification of the dental nurse assistant
- date of the operation
- premedication
- age and weight
- pre-operative assessment
- vascular access
- airway access
- drugs administered, including time and batch identification
- monitoring devices and a record of measured parameters throughout the operation
- intraoperative notes.

A dentist who carries out treatment under general anaesthesia or sedation without ensuring that the conditions set out above are fulfilled would almost certainly be considered by the General Dental Council to have acted in a manner which constitutes serious professional misconduct.

Hospital and specialist referrals

Referral for further advice, treatment or a second opinion is a responsibility of the practitioner when accepting a patient for treatment. Dentists assume a duty of care which includes the obligation to refer the patient for further professional advice or treatment, if they feel that the task in hand is beyond their own skills. If a patient is unhappy about treatment provided and requests a referral for a second opinion, you are under an obligation to comply with the request.

The referral should include the relevant demographic information on the patient as well as the clinical details. The demographic information which is required to meet the present United Kingdom hospital requirements laid down by the Department of Health should include:

- patient's name
- address, including post code
- telephone number, if appropriate
- date of birth
- name and address of dental practitioner
- name and address of medical practitioner
- National Health Service number
- religion.

The clinical details should concisely describe the problem and the treatment that has been undertaken so far. However, the 'please see and treat' referral is not acceptable. The minimum requirements should include:

- the present complaint or problem
- the history of the complaint
- the treatment provided to date
- any relevant medical history
- any relevant radiographs (with a request for their return)
- any relevant study casts
- any charting (of probing depths, for example).

In addition the following would be helpful to the specialist:

- the urgency of the referral (routine or urgent)
- the need or otherwise for an ambulance
- the preferred attendance times.

Figure 1.1. shows a specimen referral form that has been found useful. It contains all the minimum data set requirements of the Department of Health. In addition, the spaces for the hospital address and the space for the acknowledgement are arranged to fit into a modern window envelope.

Control of cross-infection

The avoidance of cross-infection in dental practice is very important, as the health of patients should not be put at risk as a result of being treated. It is the responsibility of all dental staff to ensure the absolute safety of all others working in the same environment, and the purpose of this section is to outline working methods aimed at reducing the risks of cross-infection. We must have a clear understanding of safe procedures in the avoidance of cross-infection. An essential element in the prevention of cross-infection is the competent taking of case history.

Personal protection

All clinical dental staff are strongly advised to be vaccinated against Hepatitis B and to be tested on a regular basis for an appropriate level of protective antibody. Eye protection and masks should be worn when the operator has a cold or a recurrent cold sore, and their use is also highly recommended when polishing or when creating an aerosol. Reusable or disposable gowns, laboratory coats or uniforms should be worn during clinical work, and should be changed when soiled with blood. Clinical clothes should not be worn outside clinical areas, especially where food or drink is being consumed.

Hand hygiene

At the start of each session all jewellery, wrist watches, rings and bracelets should be removed. Hands should be thoroughly washed and dried with a liquid soap, and any cuts covered with waterproof sticking plasters. The hands should then be disinfected with an alcohol-based hand-disinfectant, such as Hibisol, and allowed to dry. A new pair of rubber gloves should be worn for each patient treated. Latex gloves should be used for all procedures except where operators are sensitive to the material, when low-allergen gloves may be worn. It should be noted that rubber gloves are flammable, and great care should be exercised when carrying out any procedure which involves the use of a naked flame. Safe methods of heating, such as the 'Safe-Air' (Figure 1.2.), should be used when heat is required.

When gloves are changed between patients, the hands do not need to be rewashed if not soiled, but should be disinfected with the alcohol-based disinfectant. If non-sterile gloves are used, this procedure should also be applied to the outer surface of the gloves after they are donned. Readers are referred to the excellent paper edited by Field published in the *British Dental Journal* (Field, 1994), for further advice on hand care.

To permit effective hand-washing, taps in the surgery should be capable of being operated by the elbow or the foot or electronically, without being touched by the hands, either gloved or ungloved. Disposable towels should be used if possible.

Needlestick injuries

The most dangerous injuries in the surgery are needlesticks, and great care should be taken to avoid them. A similar injury may be caused mechanically by the tip of a scaler when it is left on the handpiece after use. In the unfortunate event of a penetrating or needlestick injury the following procedures should be adopted:

- Wash the injury thoroughly with soap under running water without scrubbing, and allow it to bleed profusely. Apply Betadine and cover, if necessary, with a suitable dressing. Check the medical

PATIENT REFERRAL LETTER

PRACTICE DETAILS

Name of referring practitioner if different from practice stamp:

....

Telephone number ....

Date ....

To: Name of Hospital
Address
City + post code

Please arrange for my patient to see:

.... (Consultant)

In the Department of ....

For: Advice / Treatment

Routine / Urgent

Transport required: YES / NO

Fold here———————————————————————————

PATIENT DETAILS (Referral details overleaf)

Title: Mr/Mrs/Miss/Ms/Other

Surname ____________________

Forenames____________________

D.O.B. ____________________

Tel. no.

Home ____________________

Work ____________________

Address

____

____

____

Post Code ____________________

Medical (or Dental if applicable) Practitioner's name and address ....

....

NHS Number ....

Religion ....

Fold here ———————————————————————————

ANY HOSPITAL

ACKNOWLEDGEMENT

PRACTICE DETAILS

❑ We have placed .... on our waiting list.

❑ An appointment has been made for ....

❑ An appointment will be sent in approximately .... weeks

CONSULTANT ....

Clinic ....

Reference no. ....

Date ....

Figure 1.1 A specimen referral form.

REFERRAL DETAILS

Reason for Referral

Relevant medical or dental history

Preferred Attendance times (Day /morning/afternoon) ....

Enclosures

(Please include recent radiographs and study models if appropriate. These will be returned after perusal)

Signature ....

PLEASE DO NOT WRITE BELOW THIS LINE

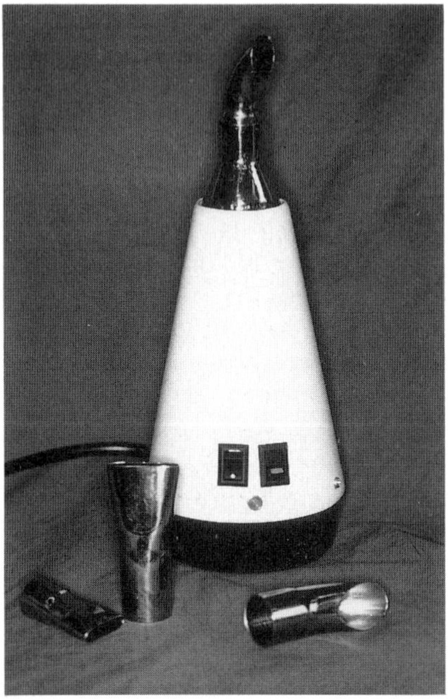

Figure 1.2 The 'Safe-Air' heater.

status of the patient concerned, and complete an accident form if appropriate.

- Where the injury has been caused by a sharp from an identified infection-risk patient, advice should be sought from the local public health laboratory. In addition, advice may often be obtained from the Occupational Health Department of a hospital. If the injured person is not immune and the patient is Hepatitis B positive, 5 ml of immunoglobulin must be given intramuscularly within 48 hours. The injured person should be followed up and given a Hepatitis B vaccination course starting within one month.

Eye protection

Spectacles must be worn by the patient and should be worn by all clinical dental staff when scaling, polishing, root planing or using ultrasonic, air scalers or air turbines.

Sterilization

Sterilization is achieved by autoclaving or with dry heat using an open tray system, and these must be the methods of choice for all non-disposable instruments after the removal of debris. Every effort should be made to use disposable items. Instruments or items of equipment which cannot be autoclaved can be disinfected by immersing in 2 per cent glutaraldehyde solution for 30 minutes or 1 per cent sodium hypochlorite for 10 minutes. Autoclaves should be checked for efficient sterilising on a regular basis.

Handpieces and air scalers must be lubricated and autoclaved after each patient and the heads of conventional handpieces should be removed before autoclaving. This lubrication is essential to prevent damage to the handpiece's internal mechanism during autoclaving. Before a sterile handpiece or air-scaler is attached to its tubing the foot switch should be activated and the water supply flushed through into the spittoon for 20 seconds to remove any organisms present in the tubing.

Sharps

All sharp instruments, whether used or not, **must** be disposed of in a 'sharps bin'. As well as obvious items such as needles, scalpel blades, suture needles and local anaesthetic cartridges, this also applies to steel burs and polishing cups and brushes. 'Sharps bins' must be sealed and replaced when not more than two-thirds full to avoid accidental injury to persons handling them.

Disinfecting dental equipment

The bracket table handle, the light switch and the light handle should not be touched when hands are contaminated, and these surfaces should be wiped with a cloth and detergent solution or sprayed with a disinfectant spray between patients and then dried, as should the working surface of the bracket table. The dry bracket table should be covered with clean paper before receiving instruments for the next patient. Tray systems should be used wherever possible. When any of the above are visibly contaminated with blood they should be wiped with a 1 per cent sodium hypochlorite solution and then dried. If, after flushing, a spittoon is visibly contaminated with blood, it should be wiped with 1 per cent sodium hypochlorite solution.

Triple syringe tips should be removed and autoclaved after the treatment of each patient. Before the treatment of the next patient, the syringe should be flushed with water for 20 seconds before an autoclaved tip is reattached. Tubing leading to handpiece or airscaler attachments and the aspirator, if not in a PVC material, should be covered with a disposable plastic sleeve fastened in place with adhesive tape to the air motor, to allow changing of sterile handpieces before surgical procedures or root planing are carried out. This or the PVC tubing should be sprayed with a disinfectant between each patient. Aspirator tubing should be flushed through with 1 per cent sodium hypochlorite solution at the end of each day.

Working practices

Heavy-duty rubber gloves must be worn by personnel cleaning operative areas or when cleaning contaminated instruments before autoclaving. Aerosol dispersal must be kept to a minimum by using a wide-bore aspirator whenever possible. When an airscaler or ultrasonic scaler is to be used, the patient should rinse with a 0.2 per cent chlorhexidine solution (e.g.Corsodyl, SmithKline Beecham, Brentford, UK) for 1 minute before treatment is started, to reduce the number of oral organisms and thereby minimize the aerosol's microbial burden.

All rotary instruments should be cleaned, ideally in an ultrasonic bath, or failing that, using a bur cleaner, and then sterilized by hot air oven. Steel burs generally should be considered as disposable, with the exception of acrylic burs.

Hands should be washed before and after using X-ray apparatus, pulp testers, bur changers and similar equipment, as well as before and after handling patient notes. Where practical, auxiliary equipment should be wiped with a cloth moistened with disinfectant solution. Bur changers are a potential source of cross-infection, and must be autoclaved between each patient.

Disinfectant solutions

Sodium hypochlorite solution

Fresh aqueous solutions of sodium hypochlorite (bleach) are recommended for general surface disinfection, as 1 per cent sodium hypochlorite solution represents 10 000 ppm available chlorine, and can be used for wiping surfaces contaminated with visible blood and for disinfection of items of equipment.

Glutaraldehyde solution

This is very toxic and should be used in a fume cupboard: 2 per cent solution activated within the past 14 days is stipulated.

Disinfectant sprays

Sprays of 0.5 per cent chlorhexidine gluconate in 70 per cent alcohol or methylated spirit are considered suitable for surface disinfection.

Further reading

BDA (British Dental Association) Advisory Service (1993a). *Health and Safety Law for Dental Practices.* Advice Sheet A3. British Dental Association, London.

BDA (British Dental Association) Advisory Service (1993b). *The control of cross-infection.* Advice Sheet A12. British Dental Association, London.

British Dental Association (1988). *Guide to blood borne viruses and the control of cross infection in dentistry.* The Association, London.

Croser, D. and Chipping, J. (1989). *Cross infection control in General Dental Practice – a practical guide for the whole dental team.* Quintessence Publishing, London.

Expert Advisory Group on AIDS (1990). *Guidance to clinical health care workers: protection against infection with HIV and Hepatitis viruses. Recommendations of the Expert Advisory Group on AIDS.* HMSO, London.

Field, E. A. (ed.) (1994). Hand hygiene, hand care and hand protection for clinical dental practice. Recommendations of the European Panel for Infection Control in Dentistry. *British Dental Journal*, **176**, 129–34.

General Dental Council (1993). *Professional conduct and fitness to practise.* The Council, London.

Wake, M. J. C. (1993). Report on 'Medicolegal Issues': Faculty of Dental Surgery (supplement). *Annals of the Royal College of Surgeons (England) Bulletin*, **75**, 156–61.

2

Conservation and fixed prosthodontics

Simon Northeast

Introduction

This chapter covers the diagnosis and primary management of problems caused by failure of restored single teeth and fixed prostheses. Not all urgent calls from patients require immediate treatment; but this is often difficult to determine, and in most cases it is essential to examine the patient as soon as possible to make a diagnosis and evaluate treatment needs. Prejudging the needs and condition of patients is all too easy, so it is essential that all dental staff offer a sympathetic and reassuring approach when dealing with restorative emergencies.

Emergencies and complications requiring operative dental care are unfortunately common. Problems range from minor chipping of teeth or restorations to major failures of large fixed prostheses. The introduction of new materials and techniques during the last decade has altered the management of operative emergencies. New adhesive methods allow repair of a greater number of failed restorations rather than replacement, thus simplifying and reducing the time spent on emergency treatment. Management of failed modern adhesive restorations may be inappropriate where knowledge and understanding of these new techniques are lacking: for example, eugenol-based temporary materials will interfere with the setting of resin luting agents and dentine bonding systems.

Primary assessment

First assess the nature of each restorative emergency and determine a short-term prognosis before planning any treatment. Information given over the telephone helps when preparing for an emergency appointment, allowing time for thought about the approach to be used when the patient visits. There are three broad types of restorative emergency: acute, sub-acute and aesthetic. Acute emergencies frequently involve pain or infection, commonly associated with pulp or periapical pathology. They require immediate treatment to alleviate suffering or to prevent spread of infection and further debilitation. Sub-acute conditions, such as broken teeth or restorations, require less urgent treatment, because they are not so threatening, but may need urgent attention to reassure concerned patients. Aesthetic emergencies involving anterior crowns or bridges are upsetting for most patients, especially when the restorations have been fitted recently. This often creates a demand for urgent treatment. Pain is not usually associated with these conditions, but delaying treatment can produce embarrassment and restrict social activity.

An increasing awareness among patients of aesthetic dental treatment has raised their expectations, and it is reasonable to expect primary emergency treatment to reflect these concerns by using high-quality aesthetic materials and appropriate techniques. There is a need to balance the patients' perceptions of their problems with the clinical findings and possible treatments. A careful history and examination is mandatory, as this may reveal important details that affect treatment planning and prognosis. Emergency care must relate to the demands of the patient and the time available for immediate treatment.

Fractured or lost restorations

One of the most common restorative problems is partial or complete loss of a restoration. This can present either simply as a technical failure or in association with recurrent caries. In either case it is often an unexpected problem, with no history of trauma. Unlike cracked tooth syndrome, it is usually easy to diagnose when part of the restoration is missing; but a retained fractured segment can make this more difficult. Loss of an anterior restoration usually prompts an early request for treatment, whereas failures in posterior teeth may go unnoticed for some time. Patients may complain of pain following exposure of dentine or discomfort from rough or sharp edges left by a loss of restorative material. Even where the restoration is merely loose, the affected tooth may hurt during chewing. For example, proximal segments of failed posterior restorations can traumatize underlying gingival tissue when displaced. Food packing may occur where failure results in loss of proximal contact. This may also lead to severe periodontal trauma and pain.

Temporary restorations in posterior teeth

Management of failed restorations depends upon the severity of symptoms. In most cases the problem is not urgent, and is best managed at a routine appointment. If the case requires immediate care a simple temporary restoration is adequate. It is important to assess the condition of any remaining restoration and check the extent of recurrent caries before planning a repair. If the retained part of a failed restoration is not undermined by caries and is self-retentive there is no need to remove the old material before placing the temporary repair. When the temporary is eventually replaced with a permanent material, retaining part of the old restoration preserves tooth tissue and simplifies the repair. Choose a temporary material that lasts until the next appointment. Do not use weak materials like zinc oxide and eugenol when a temporary restoration has to last for several weeks. The purposes of the temporary repair are to protect dentine and pulp, stabilize the position of the tooth and maintain the tooth in function. However, it would be unwise to attempt replacement of missing cusps with temporary materials, as they are likely to break off, jeopardizing the integrity of the repair.

Temporary restorations in anterior teeth

In anterior teeth temporary materials also need to restore aesthetics. Glass–ionomer cements fulfil this role because they are intrinsically adhesive and relatively simple to use. The recent introduction of glass–ionomer/resin hybrid materials may provide a better alternative (e.g. 'Vitremer', 3M Dental Products, Loughborough, UK; 'Fuji II LC', GC, Tokyo, Japan). These materials have superior aesthetics and physical properties compared with glass–ionomer cements. They have the advantages of bulk setting and command set by visible-light curing. This combined with simple bonding procedures makes them quick and easy to use. These materials will often last for many months before requiring replacement.

Fractured teeth

Tooth fracture is another common restorative emergency. The problem may range from a small enamel chip on a posterior tooth to an anterior fracture involving the pulp. Traumatic anterior tooth fractures are most common in children, and these require urgent treatment. The most common fractures occur in restored teeth, where extensive tooth preparation and non-adhesive restorations weaken the cusps. A period of pain may precede the fracture as a crack extending into dentine develops. Extensive caries may cause the collapse of undermined enamel, leading patients to think they have 'fractured a tooth'.

Vital teeth

Fractures require careful assessment, particularly following trauma. Look for root or alveolar fractures as well as soft tissue trauma. Take a radiograph to check for root or alveolar bone fracture. Fractured teeth are often painful following fresh exposure of dentine at the fracture site. The tooth may be sensitive to heat, cold and touch immediately following the fracture, and may develop symptoms of acute pulpitis as pulp irritation continues. The development of irreversible pulpitis may demand root canal therapy; therefore it is important to diagnose the condition of the pulp – which can be difficult. Most teeth will simply suffer some increased sensitivity. Treat this condition by protecting the exposed dentine with a temporary restoration, or a dentine bonding resin where function and aesthetics are unimportant.

If the tooth does not require immediate restoration smooth any rough edges to improve comfort and place a desensitizing agent on the exposed dentine. Modern dentine bonding resins are excellent for this purpose because they effectively seal the dentine surface, preventing fluid movement through dentinal tubules. In most dentine bonding systems an acid primer removes mineral from the dentine surface, leaving a porous, collagen-rich layer. Acid priming without local anaesthetic can be very painful to the patient, because dentine permeability is increased. Do not dry the dentine excessively before applying a hydrophilic resin coupling agent. This component penetrates the collagen matrix, creating a 'resin hybrid layer'. Many of the visible-light cured dentine bonding resins have a high viscosity that produces a relatively thick layer once polymerized. This treatment can eliminate dentine sensitivity for up to three months, giving plenty of time to schedule a replacement restoration. Where dentine bonding is used in the final restoration, remember to abrade the dentine surface gently to remove any remnants of resin applied as an emergency treatment.

Cusp fracture

Fractured cusps compromise the retention of restorations, especially in heavily restored teeth. Assess the stability of any residual

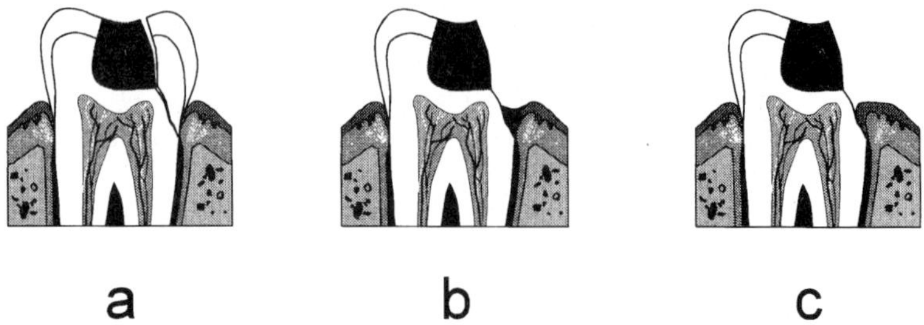

Figure 2.1 When a cusp fractures leaving a subgingival margin (a) removal of the fractured fragment causes bleeding (b) preventing adaptation of temporary materials. Where this condition is left for several days contraction of the gingivae over the fracture surface inhibits access for repair (c).

restoration. All or part of the restorations may need removal before placing a temporary. Zinc polycarboxylate or glass–ionomer cements with intrinsic adhesion to dentine reduce the need to create undercuts by removing any old material. These materials are well retained and support weakened tooth structure. When the fracture margins are supragingival a temporary is easy to place; but complications arise when an oblique cusp fracture produces a subgingival margin (Figure 2.1). The cusp may remain attached to the gingival tissue and need removing before carrying out further treatment. The resulting bleeding will inhibit identification of the fracture margins and make placement of a temporary difficult. The use of astringents such as ferric sulphate or application of localized electrosurgery usually controls bleeding for long enough to place a temporary material up to the margin of the fracture. Persistent bleeding or deep subgingival margins require surgical treatment before a final restoration is placed. This is especially likely if there has been some delay in seeking care. Under these circumstances the gingival tissue contracts during healing, restricting subgingival access to the fracture surface. When this occurs the interfering soft tissue should be removed surgically, taking into account proximity of the fracture margin to the alveolar crest. The operation is a crown-lengthening procedure, if necessary removing bone to a level 3–4 mm below the fracture line and apically repositioning the gingival crest beyond the fracture margin.

Non-vital teeth

Root canal therapy significantly weakens tooth crowns, leading to fractures. There is usually no history of pain unless the fracture causes mechanical damage to soft tissues or a vertical fracture

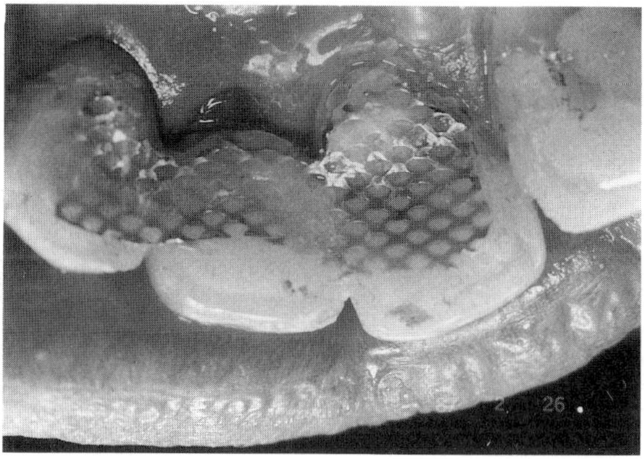

Figure 2.2 Wire mesh used to support a temporary acrylic denture tooth pontic. The mesh is bonded with visible light-cured resin composite. Reprinted courtesy of Martin Dunitz Ltd.

carries infection into the periodontal ligament. The crowns of root-filled anterior teeth restored with direct composite resin may fail by complete horizontal fracture. The resulting gap requires prompt aesthetic repair, usually with a temporary post and crown. If an accurate copy of the original contour is required and the fractured crown fragment is retained by the patient this may be secured temporarily to the root with a glass–ionomer base material and an alginate sectional impression may be taken. This is used as a matrix for constructing a resin temporary post crown that copies the original crown contour. When a fracture is deeply subgingival extract the root and construct a temporary bridge or denture to fill the gap. Alternatively, bond the extracted natural tooth crown to the adjacent teeth using etch-retained composite, or bond a denture tooth pontic using expanded wire mesh (Figure 2.2) or polymer fibre (e.g. 'Ribbond', Ribond Inc., Seattle, US) to strengthen the resin.

Non-vital root fractures

Management of root fractures in vital teeth is covered elsewhere. The most common fracture in a non-vital tooth is a vertical or

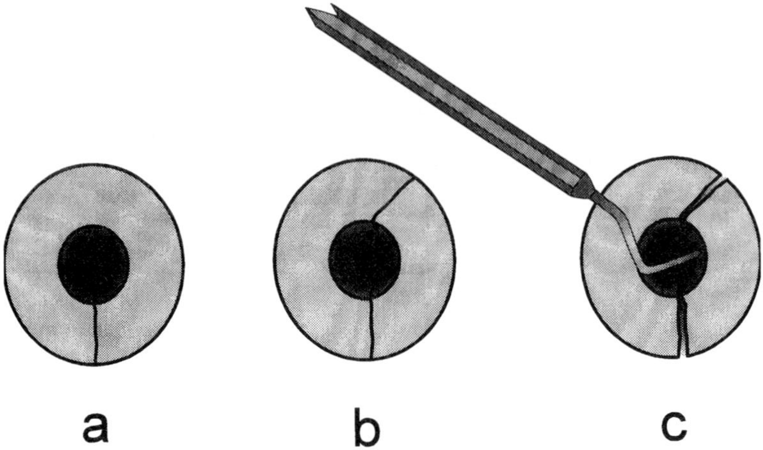

Figure 2.3 (a) Unilateral vertical root fractures show as a thin line on the root surface, and are difficult to see without magnification because the root appears intact. (b) A complete, bilateral root fracture may also be difficult to detect soon after its occurrence; but twisting an instrument in the root canal will separate the fragments, making the crack clearly visible (c).

oblique root fracture associated with a post in the root canal (Figure 2.3). A request for recementation of a loose post should always arouse suspicion that the abutment root has fractured. This may be the only sign that a fracture has occurred, because the slow spread of infection along a line of fracture may not produce symptoms for several weeks. Take care before refitting post crowns to look carefully for an incomplete, unilateral radial fracture on the root face. Gentle torque applied to the root canal may open a crack line (Figure 2.3). Magnification using binocular loupes helps the search. Another useful aid is to apply a small amount of disclosing solution or caries indicator dye to the root face. If a crack is present it will take up the dye and be seen more easily. Bilateral complete fractures are much easier to detect. The two fragments will often have separated, producing a clear gap in two places on the root face. Movement of the fragments with an instrument may be painful if a periodontal infection has developed, and pus may sometimes appear. Both conditions have a hopeless prognosis: therefore plan to extract the root and replace the lost tooth with a bridge, partial denture, or implant. Temporary cementation, or resin-bonding the old post crown, can delay extraction while constructing a temporary prosthesis.

Failed inlays and crowns

With the exception of post crowns, single-unit crowns and inlays rarely become uncemented unless the preparations lack sufficient retention. They are more likely to fail for other reasons, such as secondary caries, wear, and fracture. When inlays or crowns become uncemented they may be lost, but, if retained by the patient, can be reinstated regardless of the retention form of the preparation thanks to recently developed adhesive procedures. Like other teeth with failed restorations there is likely to be some sensitivity to hot and cold as well as discomfort during chewing. Most inlays and crowns restore occlusal function, so it is important to replace them urgently, or else the occlusion becomes unstable and deranged. The affected tooth may drift mesially and over-erupt, making refitting impossible or future restoration difficult.

Assessment and repair

Where the original restoration is lost a new temporary is required. These may vary from simple ready mixed temporary materials for a small occlusal inlay cavity to customized resin crowns for anterior teeth. Inform the patient if new caries has developed, and remove the caries before placing a temporary restoration. Make a similar check before recementing an old restoration. The patient must be informed when caries has damaged the preparation margin, and the dentist must discuss whether a new restoration is indicated. Some patients cannot immediately afford to have a new crown or inlay made. Under these circumstances, following excavation of caries, restore the defects with radio-opaque glass–ionomer cement (e.g. 'Base Line', Dentsply, Weybridge, UK; 'Ketac Bond', Espe, Knutsford, UK) or with light-cured glass–ionomer hybrids. These materials will give good service where plaque control and diet are satisfactory, but may be degraded in patients with high caries activity. Monitor repairs for marginal failure and maintain as necessary. If the defective preparation margin is accessible with the restoration in place it may be possible to make a repair after recementation.

Gingival tissues inflamed by poor plaque control adjacent to the failed restoration are likely to bleed during recementation. Anticipate the problem and take steps to control haemorrhage with a proprietary astringent, and retraction cord or electrosurgery if necessary. Where bleeding is uncontrolled it may not be possible to assess the extent of damage to the preparation margins. In this case secure the restoration with a temporary cement for two or three

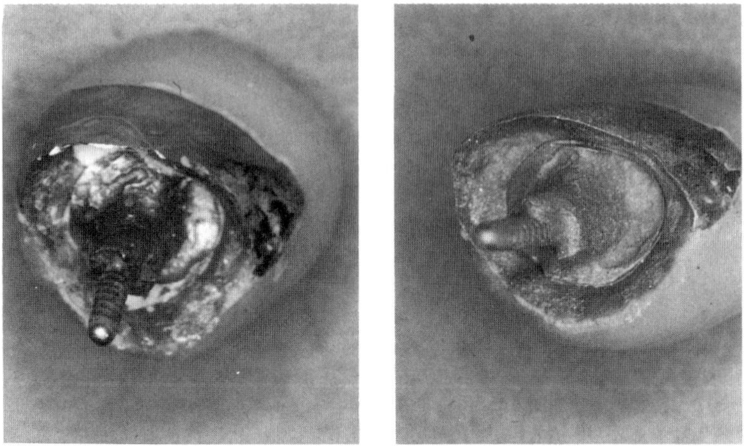

Figure 2.4 Left: The fitting surface of this uncemented post crown is covered with debris and cement, which may prevent adequate seating and inhibit good adaptation of fresh cement. Right: The same crown is shown after chairside air-blasting with 50 μm alumina grit to remove all debris and slightly roughen the surface, improving the adaptation to freshly applied cement.

days, during which time the inflammation subsides. At this time remove the crown or inlay, clean off the temporary cement and refit with a permanent cement or resin.

Recementation

Remove all the old cement from the tooth and the restoration. This is a time-consuming job with hand instruments; but a chair-side grit-blaster (e.g. 'Handi Blaster', Myron, US) makes short work of cleaning a restoration fitting surface (Figure 2.4). Extracoronal preparations are relatively easy to clean; but post holes trap food and plaque, which must be removed completely for successful recementation. A valuable aid to cleaning post holes is a small interproximal brush with a latch-fit shank for use in a slow-speed handpiece with pumice and water (e.g. 'Identobrush', Identoflex AG, Postfach, Switzerland). After cleaning away abrasive residues, reseat the restoration on the tooth preparation and evaluate the marginal fit. Previous defects such as overhangs should be recontoured within the limits of the restoration. This may be difficult on the buccal margins of porcelain fused to metal crowns, where exposed metal would show. Deal with gaps in the same way as you would for recurrent caries. Where resistance and retention form are good, the old restoration can be rapidly recemented using glass–ionomer, or zinc phosphate luting cements. For less retentive forms an adhesive luting resin may reduce the chances of recurrent failure. The tooth surfaces and restoration must be suitably prepared for a resin adhesive. Apply a low film thickness, dual-cure dentine-bonding system to the enamel and dentine (e.g. 'Mirage ABC', Myron, Kansas US; 'All Bond II', Bisco, Bisco, Itasca, US). Do not use high-viscosity light-cure dentine-bonding resins, because the thickness of the polymerized resin layer may prevent restorations from seating. There is also a risk that they may not bond well to autopolymerizing luting resins.

Metal castings should be grit-blasted with 50 µm alumina and tin-plated using a chair-side electroplater (e.g. 'Micro Tin', Danville Engineering, Danville, US) unless the alloy is known to be non-precious, in which case grit-blasting will suffice. Use a chemically adhesive resin, such as Panavia EX 21 (Kuraray Ltd, Tokyo, Japan), to bond the restoration to the tooth. This technique is also useful for cementing short posts. The difficult job of applying and drying dentine-bonding agents down a post hole is simplified by using specialized delivery systems (e.g. 'Endo Eze kit', Ultradent Dental Products, South Jordan, US). Where fit is poor, cement film thickness is not a problem, and chemically polymerized composites or glass–ionomer cement will secure an old restoration. Cleaning up the excess composite can be difficult, requiring rotary instruments. If dual-cure cements are used it is important to light-cure the margins, as these materials are highly sensitive to air inhibition when only allowed to set chemically. Light transmission to proximal margins on restorations with broad contacts is improved by using light-conducting wedges (e.g. 'Luci Wedges', Hawe Neos, Gentilino, Switzerland).

Failed temporary restorations

Temporary crowns and bridges, from their description, have limited durability. Unfortunately, they often fail prematurely, with far-reaching consequences if not repaired or replaced rapidly, so an early appointment is important. Patients must be told at the time of tooth preparation to return to the surgery if a temporary is lost before the next scheduled appointment. Loss or failure of temporary restorations can cause dentine sensitivity, drifting, over-eruption, food packing and, in anterior teeth, an embarrassing gap in a smile. Give priority to cases where an impression for the final restorations has already been taken, in order to avoid unwanted tooth movement, which would result in the need for a new impression.

Temporary restorations regularly become dislodged. When this happens and the temporary is structurally sound it should be recemented with a temporary cement (e.g. 'Temp Bond', Kerr Dental Products, Romulus, US). Thorough cleaning of the preparations and the temporary is essential for the best results. A chair-side grit-blaster rapidly removes cement from the fitting surface of temporary structures. If it is intended to use resin cements for the final restoration then **a non-eugenol-based temporary cement should be used** (e.g. Temp Bond NE, Kerr Dental Products, Romulus, US). In cases of repeated loss a more rigid material is indicated: for example, reinforced zinc oxide eugenol (e.g. Kalzinol, Dentsply, Weybridge, UK) or a polycarboxylate cement. Stronger materials, such as zinc phosphate and glass–ionomers, are contraindicated, as these may be difficult to remove, resulting in damage to the prepared tooth.

Acrylic temporaries can be repaired by brush application of new material. Light-cured composite can also be used, but this will not adhere to existing material. Where a repair is not possible a new temporary restoration is required. For single-unit preparations this can be achieved with a variety of prefabricated structures. Where a bridge is involved immediate replacement may be difficult, unless study casts or an index of the original contour are available. Where these do not exist, an alginate impression of the preparation should be cast. If fragments of the temporary bridge remain these can be used to help construct a simple wax-up. A sectional impression of the wax-up is then used as a matrix to make a new temporary bridge.

Fractured facings

General precautions

Some of the materials and techniques described in this section can be potentially harmful unless sensible precautions are taken. Organic tin-plating solutions and buffered hydrofluoric acid gels are toxic and **must not** be allowed to contact soft tissue or be swallowed. It is the writer's view that **these materials should not be used unless a rubber dam is securely fitted** over the teeth concerned to limit the area of application and thus protect the patient. Masks, gloves and eye protection must be worn by all operators when dealing with these materials. Use high-volume suction to scavenge the waste powder when grit-blasting intra-oral surfaces. Compact, illuminated dust-extraction units prevent dust contamination when grit-blasting small objects at the chair side.

Acrylic and composite

Acrylic facings on gold crowns have given way to modern composite resins, which have greater colour stability and wear resistance. While relatively few of these restorations are made, they occasionally require maintenance. Loss of acrylic facings does not result in exposure of sensitive underlying dentine, and is more of an inconvenience than a true emergency. The main problem is one of poor appearance caused by exposure of the underlying metal crown. Clean the crown with pumice and fit a rubber dam. Remove part or all of the old resin, and grit-blast briefly with 50 μm alumina, taking care to control escape of powder from the operating site. Tin-plate the metal surface using a fine-tipped wick to apply the plating solution. Wash and dry the plated surface and apply a metal primer: for example, B and C resins from Mirage ABC (Myron, Kansas, US). Apply and polymerize a thin layer of light-cured opaque resin, followed by a good-quality composite resin chosen to match the shade of the neighbouring teeth.

All-porcelain restorations

The growing provision of aesthetic ceramic veneers, crowns and bridges inevitably increases the number of failures. The high cost of replacing these restorations prompts the need for effective repair. Early techniques for repairing ceramic using silane coupling agents met with limited success. Durable results can now be achieved thanks to the recent introduction of ceramic etchants. The range of problems likely to be seen extends from small chips of porcelain to large fractures and complete loss of restorations. Patients are likely to seek help, because ceramic fractures leave a rough surface and look unattractive.

The type of retention employed will determine to what extent a fractured all-ceramic restoration may be repaired. Cemented crowns have a poor prognosis once fractured, and simple palliative treatment should be given as an emergency measure. Glass–ionomer cement should be used to replace any missing fragments of ceramic, and a new appointment should be made to remake the crown. Resin-bonded ceramic veneers, crowns and inlays are usually securely bonded to the underlying tooth. Complete debonding is likely to result from a technical error. Should this occur with a ceramic veneer then the emergency treatment will depend upon the wishes of the patient. If the change in appearance is acceptable then rough edges should be smoothed and the veneer should be remade at a later date. If temporary coverage is indicated, remove residual luting resin to expose a small region of enamel in the centre of the preparation and etch with 30–40 per cent phosphoric acid. Adapt a suitable shade of composite resin over the etched region to recontour the affected tooth, cure and polish. The temporary composite veneer is easily removed and rebonded at the scheduled appointment to remake the final restoration.

Large pieces of fractured ceramic may be rebonded to the tooth. Determine the completeness of the retained fragments by trying them on the tooth. All residual resin must be removed from the preparation and porcelain. A chair-side grit-blaster is the method of choice; alternatively, rotary instruments can be used on the tooth and the ceramic pieces can be heated to burn off the resin. Etch the enamel with 30–40 per cent phosphoric acid and the ceramic with a hydrofluoric acid (HF), or acidulated phosphate fluoride gel (e.g. 'Porcelain etch', Myron, Kansas, US). The pieces are then bonded using a light-cured composite veneer luting resin. Where a fracture does not extend to the underlying preparation, then grit-blast the affected area, etch with HF acid gel under a rubber dam, and treat with a silane coupling agent. Apply a direct composite to restore to full contour, finish and polish.

Porcelain fused to metal

Failure of porcelain facings on metal ceramic crowns has often been regarded as a difficult restorative problem, with little choice but to replace the offending restoration. New adhesive techniques offer successful temporary and longer-term repairs. Small fractures within the ceramic can be dealt with as for all-ceramic restorations. More extensive damage inevitably exposes the underlying metal, which is often unsightly, and must be masked in any repair. Any repair must bond to both metal and ceramic unless the entire facing has been lost. Damaged surfaces must be cleaned, preferably by grit-blasting, which creates a retentive surface on any exposed metal and renders it receptive to adhesive metal primers, which should be applied immediately after cleaning. Large areas of exposed metal can be tin-plated to improve bonding. Apply a metal primer before brushing a thin layer of opaque resin over the metal. Take care not to cover the ceramic with opaque, or it will show through at the margins. After light-curing the opaque resin complete the repair, using a normal-opacity composite resin, and polish. Where the entire facing has been lost it is best to regard any resin repair as temporary and schedule an appointment either to replace the crown or to construct a new resin-bonded ceramic facing.

Bridge failures

Fractures

Fracture of ceramic accounts for a significant number of bridge failures, and this problem is covered above. Sudden failure of a bridge is usually caused by fracture of a soldered joint or the connection between pontic and retainer. This structural failure reduces support for the pontic, and may allow it to bend and traumatize the gingival tissue, causing a great deal of discomfort. This condition cannot be repaired intra-orally with any currently known materials. One day, perhaps, laser technology may offer a solution! At present, there is no alternative to removing the bridge and replacing it with a new one, because repairing the old bridge is unlikely to be successful.

Retention failure

Conventional cemented bridges

Large levering forces applied to fixed bridges during function put a great strain on the luting materials, with the result that retainers occasionally become loose. Where this occurs on a fixed–fixed design the patient may not be aware that a retainer has loosened until symptoms develop or the problem is noted at a routine inspection. There is a high risk of caries developing under the retainer once it has become loose. The pumping action on the abutment soon breaks down any residual cement, leaving the space under the retainer to become colonized with plaque. Patients sometimes describe a 'sucking' sensation around the bridge during chewing of sticky foods. There may be reports of persistent pain after eating sugar-rich foods. Severe pain is usually a result of advancing pulpitis, a consequence of advanced caries and a pointer to possible root canal therapy. There is no choice but to remove bridges suffering from retention failure as soon as possible. Where complete cement failure occurs a bridge will fall out. This poses less of a threat to the abutments, as the preparations are no longer endangered by the plaque trapped under the retainers. Patients will seek help quickly under these circumstances to have the bridge recemented.

When a bridge falls out or becomes loose the abutments and the bridge must be assessed to determine the prognosis before considering recementing the bridge. The high cost of replacing a bridge is avoided if the old bridge can be refitted. Loose bridges must first be removed before the underlying preparation can be fully examined. The techniques for this are described below. Caries and other defects should be restored where possible, and both tooth and retainer surfaces cleaned thoroughly before recementing (cf. crowns). If retention and resistance form is poor, adhesive luting materials rather than conventional cements may improve the long-term prognosis. Mechanical systems are available for salvaging loose bridges: for example, the RX911 system (Whaledent, New York, US) uses self-tapping dentine pins to lock poorly retentive bridges on to abutment teeth.

Minimal preparation bridges

Resin-retained minimal preparation bridges have a disturbingly high failure rate: up to 50 per cent of posterior designs debond within five years. The chances of a repeat failure are even higher once a bridge has been rebonded. Unilateral debonding of retainers in fixed–fixed designs can have the same disastrous rapid development of caries that is so familiar beneath uncemented conventional crown-retained bridges. Resin-bonded bridges are often prescribed for younger patients, and it is in this age group that caries is most prevalent and aggressive. Debonding occurs most commonly between the metal retainer and the composite resin, rather than between enamel and resin. The layer of resin remaining on the tooth is more durable than other crown and bridge cements, and may serve to protect the underlying enamel from carious attack.

When one retainer of a fixed–fixed minimal-preparation bridge debonds, consider removing the failed metal wing, leaving the remaining retainer(s) supporting the pontic as a cantilever design. The bridge needs no further attention (apart from polishing the cut metal), and may continue to give good service for many years. Caries in the failed abutment tooth needs restoring unless it is early, in which case take steps to remineralize the lesion. If retention is judged to be excessively compromised by losing one retainer the bridge must be removed, checked and rebonded (see below for techniques).

The principles for rebonding minimal-preparation bridges are similar to those for conventional designs. All the old resin must be removed down to sound enamel on the abutments, as the bond between old and new composite is poor. Care must be taken to minimize damage to the enamel or else the fit of the retainer will be compromised. Trial fit the bridge and inspect the adaptation of the retainers, which may be distorted. Where the fit is satisfactory the bridge may be rebonded. First remove all traces of resin and plaque from the retainers. Chair-side blasting with 50 μm alumina grit is the most effective method, taking little more than a minute to clean the entire fitting surface. The surface of non-precious alloy retainers is left perfectly prepared for bonding with chemically adhesive resin cements. Efforts to salvage previously etched metal surfaces by burning off resin and ultrasonic cleaning are less likely to be successful than blasting and re-etching – a process that takes at least 20 minutes at room temperature, or longer if referred to a laboratory. Carefully isolate the abutment teeth, acid etch the enamel correctly, and bond the refurbished bridge with a resin appropriate to the type of surface preparation carried out on the retainer.

Removing crowns and bridges

The removal of failed restorations retained by cements or resin is a regular occurrence. The ease with which a restoration is removed depends upon whether it will be reused or discarded and upon the materials used in its construction. It is prudent to take an alginate impression of at least the segment of teeth surrounding the affected crown or bridge. This may be used as an index to construct a temporary restoration once the abutment teeth have been repaired. Large bridges may play an important role in occlusion and articulation. Full arch impressions should be taken in these cases to preserve a record of the occlusal relationship and articulation. Features such as anterior contours and guidance can be copied into a new bridge. Record the shade of aesthetic restorations before they are removed, to minimize difficulties in shade matching later. Extensive characterization on a failed crown or bridge is best recorded in a photograph. Alternatively, where it is reasonably preserved, the old restoration can be returned with new working impressions. Risks associated with removing crowns and bridges include fracture of abutments, damage to adjacent teeth or restorations, and inadvertent extraction of periodontally compromised teeth. It is important to assess these risks before proceeding. There is no need to remove individual crowns from teeth to be extracted, but fixed bridges may hinder extraction.

Removing all-ceramic restorations

Porcelain jacket crowns cannot be preserved during removal, and should be cut and fractured. Cut a groove running from the buccal cervical margin into the cement layer and over the incisal edge, using a coarse dome-ended diamond bur (bladed burs are blunted rapidly by ceramics). Place a gauze square behind the crown to prevent pieces of ceramic entering the airway. Fracture the ceramic by levering a large plastic placement instrument in the groove. Resin-bonded ceramic veneers and crowns are firmly adhered to the prepared tooth, making them more difficult to remove. It is important with such cases to distinguish the underlying bonding resin from tooth tissue, to prevent overcutting. Water spray from the turbine makes this difficult, because the resin is so closely colour-matched; and so the surface must be dried frequently.

All-metal and porcelain fused to metal crowns

Both types of restoration may be removed intact, and this approach should be used before resorting to cutting. A variety of instruments are available for removing crowns and bridges (Figure 2.5). These range in complexity, from a simple sticky resin material which binds opposing teeth to complex devices that clamp the crown and apply force to adjacent teeth or to the underlying preparation through a hole made in the occlusal surfaces of the crown. Where margins are accessible a large instrument with a sharp edge may be inserted and twisted to lever the crown off. If this fails ultrasonic vibration from a periodontal scaler may help to break up the cement. Piezoelectric devices are the most powerful for this application. A popular instrument is the sliding, or spring-loaded, weight, which applies a sharp tap to the crown while continuous pressure is maintained on the crown margin. It is important to reassure patients before using these instruments, because of their frightening appearance and potentially aggressive action. Where the crown margin is well adapted to the tooth there is nowhere to apply the tips of a crown remover. In this case cut a groove in the crown to create a point of application.

When all attempts to remove a crown intact fail then it must be cut off. Gold alloys are relatively soft, and parts of a crown may be rather thick. Bladed burs cut gold alloys more efficiently than diamonds. Several patterns of specialized cross-cut tungsten carbide bur are available. These burs should be used with caution in high-torque air turbines, because they tend to chatter and break at high speed. A speed-increasing (red ring) motor-driven handpiece permits

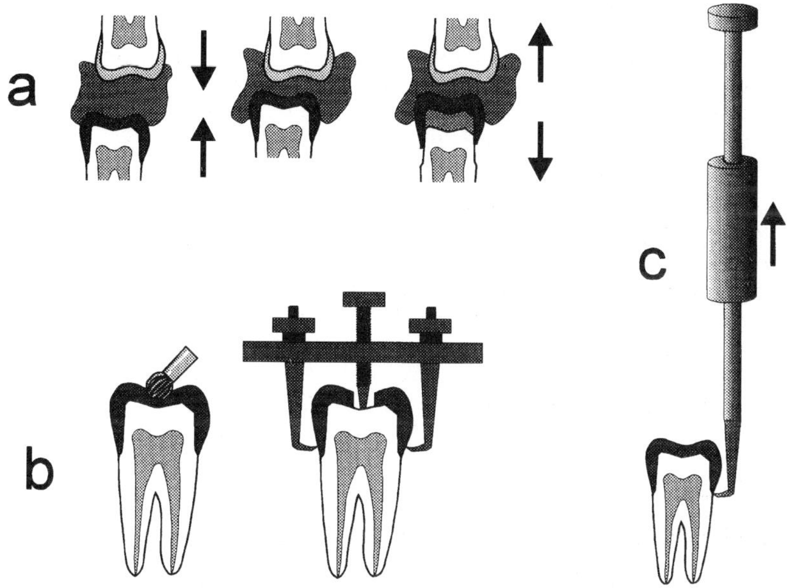

Figure 2.5 Several methods of crown removal are illustrated: (a) A sticky compound is softened by warming, placed between the teeth and closed upon. Once the material has cooled the patient is instructed to open rapidly and firmly; this usually results in removal of the crown. (b) The device shown here requires a small hole to be drilled in the occlusal surface of the crown, through which a force is applied to the underlying preparation. This is similar to a 'sprocket puller', used by automotive engineers to remove gears from shafts. (c) This popular device uses a sliding weight to apply a sharp force to the margins of a crown or bridge retainer. This technique is very successful, but depends upon a good purchase being established at the crown margin. It may be necessary to make an undercut with a bur to remove a well-fitting crown.

application of much greater pressure at lower, safer speeds, giving fast, smooth cutting. Crowns should be cut along their buccal wall through to the cement, to open a groove from the cervical margin. Twist a large straight chisel or plastic placement instrument in the cut to open out the walls of the crown. A further cut along the occlusal aspect may be required when the metal is thick. Allow more time to remove complex gold inlays, which may require several cuts and undercutting to obtain a purchase with an instrument.

Porcelain fused to metal crowns are more rigid than gold alloy crowns. When cutting off these crowns the porcelain is cut first with a diamond bur into the metal coping. Sufficient porcelain must be removed to give access to the metal and to enable the crown to flex.

The bur is changed for a cross-cut tungsten carbide, and the cut is continued through the remaining thin layer of metal to the cement. The technique for removal is the same as for gold crowns; but care must be taken to protect the airway from flying splinters of ceramic that shatter as the crown is distorted.

Removing posts and cores

Occasionally the root filling in post crowned teeth fails, and may require urgent treatment. The traditional treatment is an apicectomy; but current opinion prefers an orthograde approach. The crown, post and core have to be removed to access the canals. When remaking crowns and bridges previous posts may be judged to be too short or may suffer other defects. They must be renewed before constructing the final restorations. The technique for removing a post depends on how it is retained in the root canal. Close examination of a pre-operative radiograph will show whether the post is a threaded design, such as a Dentatus screw, Kurer post or Radix anchor, or a cast smooth-sided post. Confusion may occur with serrated designs like the Parapost, which is cemented and not screwed into place. Before attempting to remove a post the crown or bridge should be removed, often with the post where it is short or loose.

Threaded posts must be unscrewed from the root. On no account should attempts be made to pull the post directly out, as this may risk fracturing the root. Each threaded design has its own method of anti-rotation applied to the root face: for example, a lock nut on Kurer posts. Once the anti-rotation feature is removed the post can be turned anti-clockwise to unscrew it from the canal. Fine root-extraction forceps are applied to the post and twisted. Take care not to apply excessive force, especially if the neighbouring abutment has been anaesthetized. If the post cannot be loosened try applying an ultrasonic device to the post to help break up the cement. If this fails then a Masserann kit (see below) is required to cut a collar of dentine round part of the post until it can be freed by further twisting. Should this become necessary, the core diameter must be reduced to that of the post, otherwise an excessively large cylinder will be cut by the Masserann trepan bur. Other prefabricated posts may be loosened by twisting and then pulling, either with forceps or by using a special post crown remover which applies a reciprocal force to the root face, not the periodontal ligament (Figure 2.6). An anti-rotation key-way is frequently constructed in cast posts; so twisting these may result in a fractured root. This design must be removed by pulling along the path of insertion.

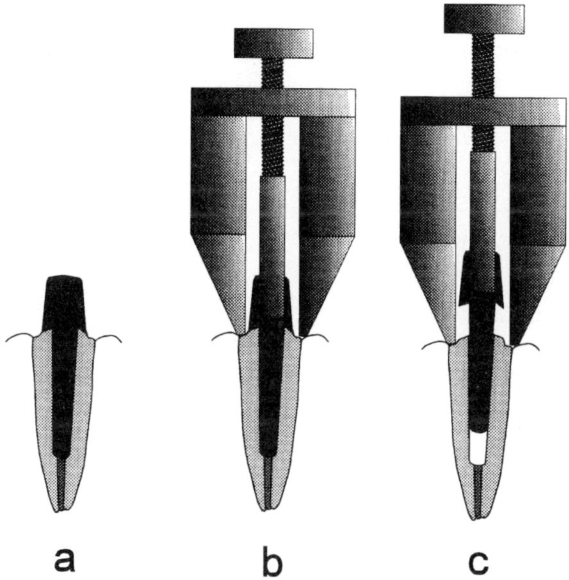

Figure 2.6 Cemented dowel posts are difficult to remove, because they are small and their margins are inaccessible to crown removers. Most post pullers depend upon reciprocal forces being applied between the post and the root face, thus avoiding applying excessive force to the periodontal ligament. The central element of the device grips the post firmly, and the two outer 'legs' rest on the root face (b). The post is withdrawn by turning a thumbscrew (c).

Removing fractured posts

Porosity or other weakness in a post and core may sometimes cause the post to fracture. When this happens the proximal part of the post remains in the root, often with little or no extension beyond the root face. No attempt should be made to cut out a fractured metal post with burs. The post is much harder than the surrounding tooth tissue, causing burs to drift into the root and risk lateral perforation. Where excessive post preparation has weakened the root then retrieval of the remnants will produce a very poor prognosis, and the root will require removal and probably prosthetic replacement.

Where sufficient width of root dentine remains a Masserann kit (Micro Mega, Lyon, France) must be used to retrieve the retained fragment (Figure 2.7). The kit contains a range of thin, end-cutting cannulae (trepan burs) of different overlapping diameters. It is also used to remove broken endodontic instruments and silver points from root canals. The kit is expensive, and must be used carefully

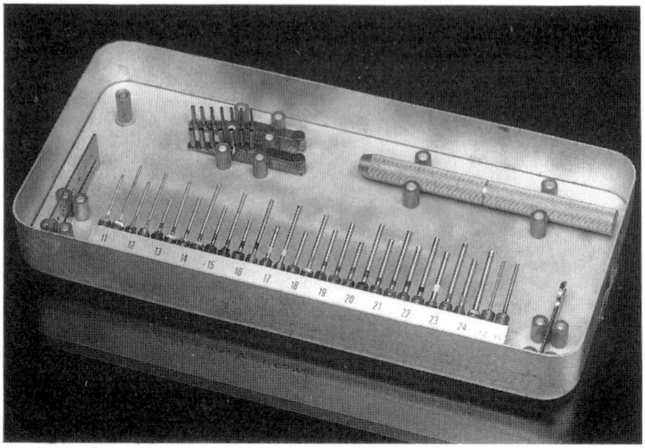

Figure 2.7 A Masserann kit comprising cylinder gauges, trepan burs and handle.

to avoid damaging the cannulae by applying excessive force. A gauge is supplied to help select the correct size of cannula, which is chosen to be a fraction wider than the post. This is rotated anti-clockwise in a hand chuck around the post, which guides the instrument as it removes a thin cylinder of dentine with minimal risk of lateral perforation. Cutting depth should be gauged against a periapical radiograph. After progressing to a significant depth the next smallest size of cannula is used to grip the broken post, twisted and pulled (Figure 2.8). This is repeated as necessary until the fragment is recovered. Once the root canal is clean a temporary post crown can be constructed.

Removing bridges

Techniques used to remove bridges differ, depending on the desired outcome of treatment. A bridge may be removed intact where the abutment teeth are sound and the bridge has simply debonded. When one or more abutment teeth or bridge sections have failed the affected retainer should be cut off. The remaining retainer(s) can be removed intact to preserve part of the bridge, or carefully cut, avoiding damage to the preparations. In some complex cases part of a bridge may be left in situ after sectioning the failed component. Sectioning may also help to remove large bridges. Treatment plans using complex bridges should include design elements that allow sections that have an increased risk of failure to be removed. Simple movable attachments are the most common method of breaking up a complex design. These enhance durability by reducing stress on pier abutment retainers.

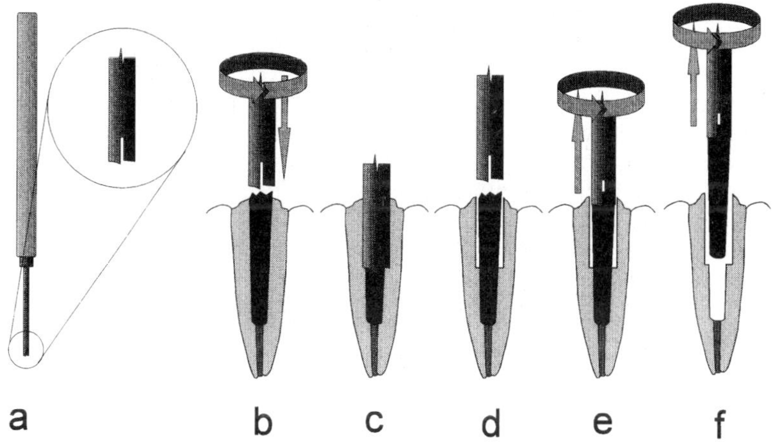

Figure 2.8 This diagram illustrates the action of a Masserann trepan bur in removing a fractured post. The tip of a Masserann trepan bur is shown in detail (a). A trepan is chosen with an internal diameter that just fits over the fractured post (b). This is applied to the root surface and rotated **anti-clockwise**, using the handle provided or in a speed-reduction contra-angle handpiece (c). The trepan must be removed frequently to allow cutting debris to be cleared, until a sufficiently deep cylinder of dentine has been cut (d). A radiograph will assist in determining this depth. A slightly narrower trepan is then selected that grips the fractured end of the post, which is turned anti-clockwise and pulled at the same time (e). It may be necessary to deepen the cut before the post is retrieved (f).

Cemented, crown-retained bridges

Most bridges, except minimal-preparation resin-bonded bridges, can be removed intact by subjecting them to sharp forces along their path of insertion. The junction between pontic and retainer forms a convenient, safe location for applying force to remove a bridge. Choose the appropriate-shaped interchangeable tip to fit under a crown margin or into an embrasure area. Sharp firm taps delivered by a sliding or spring-action crown and bridge remover usually manage to break the cement lute. Several precautions need to be taken when using these instruments. Tie a long piece of floss firmly round the bridge to protect the patient in case the bridge falls to the back of the mouth. The tip of the bridge remover must be held firmly in place while maintaining a reasonable pull along the path of withdrawal. Where one retainer is already loose the load should be applied close to the opposite retainer, otherwise large torquing forces could fracture the abutment.

Another technique for removing bridges intact uses a loop of soft stainless steel wire passed through an embrasure on the pontic. The loop may be tensioned either with a sliding-weight device as described above, or with a heavy pair of wire-bending pliers. The wire must be tight, or it will spring and absorb the shock of any force applied. The procedure is uncomfortable and can be frightening, so patients must be told what to expect and given the chance to decline, preferring instead to have their bridge cut off and replaced. A successfully removed intact bridge should be assessed along with its abutments before recementing (see elsewhere in this chapter). Parts of the bridge may be used in conjunction with new components soldered or connected via attachments.

Resin-bonded, minimal preparation bridges

The relative flexibility of minimal-preparation wing retainers permits them to be peeled off the abutment teeth. A straight chisel applied to the margin of a retainer and tapped with a mallet will readily remove anterior bridges. The sliding-weight instruments for removing conventional crowns and bridges also work well on resin-bonded bridges. Some clinicians advocate ultrasonic instrumentation to help break the resin bond. The main difficulty in removing resin-bonded metal wings is finding a niche or undercut in which to apply the instruments. To overcome this problem an inverted cone tungsten carbide bur will remove a feathered edge on a retainer margin, creating a ledge on which to apply an instrument. Thick retainers will be the most difficult to remove, because of their stiffness, and these may need sectioning. New tungsten carbide burs cut much faster through nickel–chromium alloys than diamonds. Do not compromise future retention by careless removal of enamel.

Precision attachments

The large variety of precision attachments in current use precludes consideration of individual designs in this book. Manufacturers have specific guidelines for the repair and maintenance of each type, and the reader is referred to these for specific cases. Problems that are likely to be encountered as emergencies include wear, fracture and abutment failures.

There are two broad uses of attachments: connections for fixed prostheses and retainers for removable prostheses. Those used in semi-fixed bridges provide limited stress-breaking movement around the joint and are not affected by serious wear. They rarely cause problems; on the contrary, careful use of dovetail joints in complex bridge designs facilitates easy sectional maintenance should a posterior segment of a bridge require repair or remaking. It is recommended that the female part of an attachment is located on the distal aspect of the mesial retainer or pier abutment. Should the distal segment fail it can be easily removed and a new section made or modified from a new impression. The dovetail slot is easily recorded in an impression; but when poured in stone the attachment is extremely fragile. To overcome this problem a manufactured dummy male component is inserted in the female attachment and picked up with the impression. Where a commercial dummy attachment is not available an acrylic one can be constructed directly in the mouth. The dummy is later incorporated in the wax pattern for the new distal bridge segment.

Greater and more frequent problems are encountered where attachments are used to support and retain removable dentures. Emergency problems are likely to result from sudden retention failure caused by fracture or loss of key components such as springs, studs, caps or magnets. Diminished retention resulting from gradual wear of attachments is more likely to be mentioned by a patient during routine recall appointments. In ageing prostheses there is a progressive loss of vertical dimension as the denture and natural teeth wear. This can expose parts of the attachments that secure them to the prosthesis. When this occurs the attachment rapidly becomes loose and suddenly fails. There is little that can be done in these cases, except perhaps to gain more time by refitting the attachment using self-cure acrylic and temporarily raising vertical dimension by adding a layer of acrylic to the occlusal surfaces of the prosthesis. The long-term solution is likely to involve increasing the vertical dimension or doing away with attachments in favour of a simple removable partial denture. It is unreasonable to expect many practitioners to carry a range of spare parts to repair failed attachments. Advice to the patient about using denture fixatives may help until new parts can be fitted. Technical description of repairs is beyond the scope of this chapter, but the principles are similar to the technique described above for repairing semi-fixed bridges, irrespective of whether the attachments are intra- or extra-coronal.

Crowns and bridges supporting attachments occasionally become loose. The restoration should be removed and assessed as described above. Where feasible the retainer or bridge should be recemented, even temporarily if this maintains function and appearance. Perhaps of more serious concern is extraction of an attachment abutment, particularly when this is near the front of the mouth. It is best in these cases to delay extraction until a new temporary prosthesis has been made. Attention should be directed at relieving pain, controlling infection and restoring large defects or cement failure, to retain function and await arrival of the temporary prosthesis.

3

Removable prosthodontics

David J Lamb

Complete dentures

Problems with complete dentures are common, and many demand urgent treatment. When classifying these problems it is best to divide them into three types, viz., those which new patients may complain about on their first visit to the surgery, those which the operator becomes aware of during treatment, and those which cause problems at the review stage. While not all problems fall exclusively under one of these headings, use of the classification is helpful in order to avoid repetition.

Problems from new patients

Following a period of satisfactory service from their dentures, the commonest problem patients have that requires urgent treatment is pain. If patients do not have this complaint, then no irreversible changes should be made to their dentures, lest the treatment be unsuccessful and pain result. The patients will then be unable to wear their dentures until new sets are made. This is particularly important when changes in face height are contemplated.

Other problems which require treatment, the urgency for which which will be significantly influenced by the patient's own expectations, are lack of security, nausea, changed appearance and fracture. Finally there are denture stomatitis and angular cheilitis, patients with a sensitivity to the components of denture base, and patients complaining of burning mouth.

Pain

This is a common complaint, for which immediate treatment is required. For new patients the usual underlying cause is alveolar resorption, which proceeds inexorably from the time the teeth are extracted. No denture maintains its original good fit for other than a relatively short period of time – a period of time which is particularly brief following insertion of immediate dentures. As a consequence of the different patterns of resorption, the approaches to pain from the mandible and maxilla differ, and may be dealt with separately. Rarely, a fault in the denture may cause temporomandibular joint (TMJ) pain.

Maxillary denture

Resorption of the maxillary alveolus is normally much less than that of the mandible. Nevertheless, significant loss does occur, and the resulting poor fit results in excess pressure locally. Pain, redness and ulceration occur either at the periphery (often in the region of the zygomatic process of the maxilla, where only thin mucosa separates the denture border from a near-horizontal shelf of bone), or over the midline of the palate (a zone of non-alveolar bone which is resistant to resorption). In either case the related part is reduced. Care should be taken to review progress, for fear the pain and inflammation are indicative of an expanding lesion rather than pressure from a denture.

Mandibular denture

Resorption is much more rapid in the mandible, and pain due to an ill-fitting denture tends to occur earlier. Again, the first concern is to provide relief by reducing the denture. However, because resorption is more generalized, relief of one area tends to be followed by pain recurring elsewhere; and if new dentures are to be made it is better to prevent further pain over the next few weeks (and at the same time resolve any inflammation and swelling that might compromise the accuracy of the impressions) by lining the fitting surface of the denture with a soft liner.

After cleaning and drying the denture and applying lubricant as appropriate, sufficient soft liner is mixed so that, after lining the denture, a continuous intact layer is produced. If the denture shows through or the layer of soft lining is less than 1–2 mm thick (test the thickness with a sharp probe), a further addition is made. When inflammation has resolved, working impressions can be made and new dentures constructed.

With extreme loss of alveolar bone, pain can be the result of abrasion of the denture bearing area by constant movement of the unstable lower denture (especially when there is some degree of hyposalivation), or alternatively due to pressure on the mental nerve. While wide relief of the denture over the mental foramen can help in the latter case, the former is more difficult to treat (and made worse by silicone rubber soft liners). Often only osseointegrated fixtures can give the lower denture the support and stability required to allow long-term pain-free function.

TMJ pain
It is easy to imagine TMJ pain being due to loss of face height as a result of alveolar resorption, especially when associated with protrusive over-closure. However, arthritic changes in the joints are not uncommon in elderly patients, and a radiograph of the mandibular condyle may confirm the true cause of the pain. When over-closure is thought to be the cause, vacuum-formed soft acrylic splints placed on the lower denture will temporarily increase the face height and help alleviate the symptoms. Different thicknesses can be used until the most comfortable increase is achieved, when new dentures can be made to the new face height. Permanent additions to the occlusal surface of the lower denture can be made, but the operator must be prepared for the difficulty of removing them if instead of producing benefit they cause pain from the denture-bearing area due to the change in jaw relations.

Lack of security

'Looseness' of a denture is a common complaint, and its diagnosis is further explored in the next section, where it is dealt with following insertion of the dentures. At this stage most patients accept that they must put up with the insecurity for a few more weeks until new dentures are made. Some insist on immediate correction of their complaint – perhaps for an important engagement at which they do not wish to risk embarrassment. When assessing patients under these circumstances certain common oral conditions give special problems, and the most convenient way to discuss the treatment of these is first to take cases primarily affecting either the upper or the lower jaw, and then those involving both.

Maxilla
Although alveolar resorption is less in the maxilla than the mandible, it results in a tilting of the maxillary denture, with the anterior part rotating upwards – a movement exacerbated by any fibrous replacement of the anterior alveolus. During the interval while new dentures are being made a temporary improvement in upper denture security can be made by adding a new functional post dam. Autopolymerizing reline material is beaded along the post dam region and the denture is replaced in the mouth under occlusal pressure until the addition has gelled. After polymerization is complete, any excess material is removed. When insecurity is

associated with a significant degree of fibrous replacement of the anterior maxilla, more careful assessment must be made before instituting treatment. Many cases are associated with retained, or a history of recently extracted, lower anterior teeth, through which the damaging anteriorly-directed forces thought to cause the condition have been transmitted to the maxilla. When this condition is encountered, immediate improvements in the security of the upper denture are impossible. Instead the natural teeth are best used for improving the security (and hence tolerance) of a partial lower denture. If then a lower denture can be worn with confidence, the masticatory forces will be distributed over the entire maxilla, so allowing occlusal forces to be resisted posteriorly and preventing further progress of the condition. Often, however, the retained teeth have reduced bone support and are of little use in designing conventional support for a partial denture. A complete overdenture is usually the best prescription. Removal of the abutment crowns ensures that the denture is worn!

When the lower anterior teeth have been extracted and a fibrous anterior maxilla remains, treatment is directed to providing adequate security of the upper denture despite the state of the ridge. In mild cases two-part impression techniques can be tried. After making primary casts, a working impression is taken in a close-fitting tray with a window in the anterior region over the fibrous area. Excess material is removed from the window, the tray is repositioned in the mouth and the fibrous tissue protruding through the window is recorded in a fluid silicone impression material. The alternatives are surgical. If sufficient bony ridge remains to provide resistance to antero-posterior movement of the upper denture, the fibrous tissue can be excised. Alternatively an inert biocompatible material (e.g. hydroxyapatite) may be implanted to help restore the firmness of the original tissues. In extreme cases a bone graft and later placement of osseointegrated fixtures are the treatment of choice.

Mandible

When patients demand immediate treatment for their loose lower denture an improvement can be made using temporary soft lining. A more long-lasting improvement can be made by adding a layer of chairside reline to the fitting surface, but these materials are not intended for long-term use. They tend to discolour and become brittle with time, and will not provide permanent relief.

Both jaws

When, after a period of satisfactory service, loss of security of either or both dentures is associated with no obvious fault, it is necessary to look elsewhere for the source of the problem. The elderly are frequently prescribed medication for concurrent disease, and drug-induced hyposalivation is common. Not only may hyposalivation be caused by a drug with this known side-effect, but drugs not normally recognized as having this potential may act in synergism. When hyposalivation is the cause of denture looseness, prescription of an artificial saliva can dramatically improve the situation – aerosol types are usually more acceptable.

Nausea

Less commonly in patients with a history of satisfactory service in the past, nausea is the presenting complaint. When this is a consequence of the upper denture dropping during function and contacting the dorsum of the tongue, it is sometimes possible to improve the condition immediately by adding a functional post dam in the manner described above, so increasing the security of the upper denture. Nausea in the absence of obvious dental causes may be due to gastro-intestinal disease, and a careful history must be taken and investigations should be made.

Appearance

After a period of years a complete denture wearer may complain of a reduction in face height. It is common for dentists to attempt to increase the face height with new dentures and eliminate the freeway space, so exceeding the patient's tolerance and causing pain. When there is any doubt how great an increase in face height can be tolerated by the patient it is possible to add small amounts of autopolymerizing acrylic resin incrementally to the occlusal surface of the lower denture and assess the effect of gradual increases in face height. Alternatively, to avoid permanent modification of the lower denture, a vacuum-formed soft splint can be provided.

Careful assessment is required when the complaint is of insufficient support for the facial soft tissues. With age there is a diminution in the amount of fat in the subcutaneous tissue and an increase in the depth of natural creases, which appear more marked with loss of the natural teeth. Radial lines around the lips become obvious, especially if the upper anterior teeth have been sited further lingually than the natural teeth. When purely age-related, such changes are difficult to eliminate without exceeding the patient's tolerance, and careful judgment is required before improvements can be promised. If the cause of the patient's complaint is not entirely age-related, improvements in appearance can usually be produced by changes in the position of the teeth, but less often by thickenings of the denture periphery.

Denture fracture

Before repairing a fractured denture, future treatment must be considered in the light of the reason for the fracture occurring. Fractures normally occur either as a result of an accident, or during use. If, as is very common, the fracture is the result of an accident, for example from being dropped, and the history leads you to think this may be a regular occurrence in the future, replacement of the denture by one made from an impact-resistant resin may be helpful.

A fracture may occur during function for one of two reasons. The base may be insufficiently strong: i.e., the base dimensions are not great enough or there is insufficient space between the ridges to allow an adequately thick base. Alternatively a stress-concentrating factor, such as a notch in the periphery related to a fraenal attachment, is present. In the former case, replacement of the denture by one with a cast metal base is indicated, provided that adequate attachment can be secured between the base and the acrylic superstructure. In the latter case, surgery to remove the local cause is the treatment of choice.

When the cause for the fracture has been identified and it has been decided that dentures of a more appropriate design are to be made, the fractured denture is repaired as a temporary measure to preserve appearance while the new dentures are made. There is therefore no need to ensure the longevity of the repair. Similarly, dentures made more than 2–3 years earlier are already likely to be ill-fitting, so repair should be a temporary measure while new dentures are being made.

A fracture occurring within a year or so of the dentures' being made has a different prognosis, and the repair must be expected to last for a much longer period of time. However, it is difficult to ensure that a repair has reasonable longevity unless the fractured parts are precisely located. This can never be guaranteed, so in order to ensure that congruence of the fitting surface of the denture and the denture-bearing surface is as close as possible the repaired denture should be relined. A precontact check record and remount should also be carried out to eliminate occlusal errors.

Denture stomatitis (denture-associated candidosis)

Denture stomatitis is characterized by redness and inflammation beneath the upper denture, and is caused by candidal infection. If mild and localized it must be distinguished from trauma due to an ill-fitting denture. More severe types (characterized by inflammation beneath the entire upper denture-bearing area) are consistently associated with proliferation of *Candida*. Long-lasting infections also induce papillary hyperplasia of the mucosa.

Where trauma is the cause, the denture should be adjusted and smoothed as appropriate; but treatment is more complex when *Candida* is responsible. Differential diagnosis may be made on the basis of culture of swabs. Swabs are taken of the palate, the fitting surface of the denture, and the dorsum of the tongue. *Candida* is an oral commensal, and only when large numbers of colony-forming units (CFUs) are detected on culture can candidosis be diagnosed with certainty. The underlying cause of the candidosis is usually lack of oral hygiene, and the first step in treatment is to encourage an improvement. Steeping the dentures in 1 per cent hypochlorite is a most effective therapy, but it is often difficult to persuade an elderly person of the need to change the habits of a lifetime in order to cure a disease of which he or she has little awareness. In some cases the candidosis is associated with a systemic disease, for example immunodeficiency, diabetes, anaemia, malignancy, etc., or with concurrent therapy with antibiotics, cytotoxic drugs or steroids. Where a denture-associated candidosis fails to resolve despite improvements in oral hygiene, appropriate special tests should be carried out or further enquiries made into the medical history.

When improvements in oral hygiene fail to cure the disease it may be necessary to employ chemotherapy. Local treatment with Miconazole Oral Gel is useful, but patients sometimes object to its texture. Fluconazole tablets (50 mg once daily for 2 weeks) are a systemic alternative; but unless the predisposing cause is treated, reinfection is common.

It is sometimes difficult to convince an elderly person that the condition requires treatment. However, oral candidosis can disseminate to other parts of the body, either by local spread or via the bloodstream, particularly if the immune response is deficient. Denture stomatitis should therefore always be treated promptly when detected, and the patient should be encouraged to comply with the therapeutic regime. To aid denture-cleansing routines the fitting surface of any new dentures should be as smooth and self-cleansing as possible.

Angular cheilitis

Angular cheilitis is a painful cracking at the corners of the mouth. Classically it is presumed to occur in denture wearers as a consequence of over-closure. Lack of support at the commissures of the mouth then allows maceration of the skin with saliva and subsequent infection, either by *Candida* from the mouth or by staphylococci from the skin. The infected area can crack and bleed when the patient eats and speaks.

Treatment is by prescription of an appropriate antibiotic following culture (miconazole is effective against both *Candida* and staphylococci), followed by provision of new dentures with proper support of the soft tissues. Proper support of the soft tissues does not result from drastic increases in face height. Instead, the soft tissues are supported by the correct positioning of the teeth.

Despite all efforts, complete, permanent resolution of the angular cheilitis may not follow, and the patient may need to apply an emollient protective layer (Vaseline is useful) when it recurs.

Acrylic resin allergy and monomer hypersensitivity

An allergy to acrylic resin is rare, and gives rise to redness and inflammation of all areas in contact with the denture. When suspected it can sometimes be confirmed by questioning about any reactions to textile fibres, of which *poly*methylmethacrylate is a common constituent. Eczematous changes might also be seen around hearing aids and spectacle frames. Diagnosis is usually made by patch tests, although tests on the skin do not precisely reproduce the reactions of the oral mucous membrane, and *in vitro* challenging of the patient's lymphocytes is most reliable. If acrylic resin allergy is confirmed, dentures must be made of alternative materials such as Nylon – which requires injection moulding and tends to expand with time as it absorbs water from the saliva. Injection-moulded polycarbonate is also a possibility, if a laboratory can be found which provides such a service.

Sensitivity to *mono*methylmethacrylate is much more common, and occurs when the residual monomer content of the denture is high, usually owing to use of a short denture-curing cycle to save time. The symptoms are similar to those of acrylic allergy, but there is usually a history of the symptoms beginning immediately after the current denture was made or relined. Treatment is either to make new dentures using an adequately long curing time at a high enough temperature, or to reinvest and recure the current dentures.

Burning mouth

The problem of burning mouth can be distressing for patient and operator. It is characterized by a burning or painful sensation, which may be in the palate, tongue, alveoli, or cheeks, or in all four. Three types are defined: viz., local, systemic or psychological, according to the diagnosed cause.

Local condition
Many denture faults may cause the condition, including lack of interocclusal space, insufficient tongue space, or a rough surface. Burning mouth can also occur if there is sensitivity to monomer or if salivary flow is reduced, with poor lubrication of the denture. It can be diagnosed by removal of the denture, when the symptoms are relieved. Diminished salivary flow might be suspected if there is a history of therapy with drugs having this side-effect. Enquiry should also be made of any mouth rinse or changes in denture-cleansing agent – allergy to a constituent is a possibility. Great care should be taken to eliminate all possibility of a local cause before incriminating a systemic or psychological condition.

Systemic condition
Burning mouth can be associated with anaemia, diabetes or hormonal deficiency. Appropriate special tests can be prescribed to pinpoint the problem, but treatment is not in the province of restorative dentistry, and referral to a physician or specialist in oral medicine would be the correct path to follow.

Psychological condition
Depression or cancer phobia can manifest itself as burning sensations in the mouth. While reassurance is sometimes sufficient to cure the latter condition, depression has more complex causes, and is best left to more expert hands.

Problems during denture construction

Problems at the impression stage

Nausea
Before impressions are taken patients will often warn the operator if nausea is going to be a problem. Alternatively, nausea may be suspected if the palate of the patient's upper denture has been drastically relieved. The problem is often minor, and can be overcome by a confident manner along with reassuring the patient that this is a common condition and that you are fully prepared and confident. If retching does occur, but without great distress to the patient, the patient's head is tilted downwards, forwards and to the side over the spittoon or a hand-held kidney dish into which debris and saliva

can drip. Always maintain firm control over the impression tray in the patient's mouth. Spraying topical anaesthetic over the soft palate and fauces may not help by itself, but may give psychological support by furnishing the patient with additional proof that you are being as helpful and constructive as possible. If this fails, it is likely that even if impressions were taken it would be necessary to 'condition' the patient to allow the further stages of denture construction to be carried out. Some form of training base is made first. Take impressions in a warm, viscous impression material – dental composition is ideal. The impression material must be removed fairly expeditiously and often lacks surface detail, the base requiring additions of autopolymerizing resin at the periphery at the insertion stage to secure peripheral seal and retention. The patient is then advised to try to wear the base for increasing periods of time. As an auxiliary aid a toothbrush can be used to brush the hard palate, brushing increasingly further back. A piece of sticky tape on the brush handle allows the patient to keep track of progress. Hypnotherapy is also useful to overcome this handicap. If such help is available it can be co-ordinated with use of the training base.

If the patient can finally be conditioned to wearing a training base, it is possible to proceed as normal with denture construction. When conditioning is only partial, artificial teeth can be added to the base a few at a time by means of cold-cure resin. In severe cases the final denture may consist merely of base and anterior teeth.

Problems at the registration stage

Tremor

Accurate recording of the jaw relations demands stable registration blocks and accurate measurement of rest face height. Parkinson's disease is commonly associated with both rigidity and tremor, and will make recording the jaw relations imprecise. After recording the jaw relations a free-sliding, cuspless occlusion is prescribed. Some of the drugs used in treating Parkinson's disease also cause dry mouth (not levo dopa, however) and a liquid denture fixative may be needed to stabilize the blocks.

Communication

Accurate recording of the jaw relations also demands good communication in order to encourage patients to allow their jaws to pass into the retruded position. Patients who are not fluent in the language of the operator must bring an experienced translator with them, otherwise errors will occur. Deafness is a common problem in the elderly, and is helped by slow, clear speech rather than shouting. Face the patient and allow them to use any lip-reading abilities they have developed. A person who can converse in sign language is an asset to any practice.

Problems at the insertion stage

Pain

On insertion of a denture there are two common reasons for pain. The denture base may traumatize the soft tissues when entering a bony undercut, or there may be a pimple or blemish on the fitting surface. If the cause is an undercut, pain is felt only on insertion and removal of the denture. The undercut should be removed from the base without reducing the extent of the related denture flange. It is often thought unnecessary to remove both bilateral opposed maxillary undercuts in the tuberosity region and that removing one is sufficient – the other acting to retain the denture. This is fallacious; both undercuts must be removed.

A pimple or blemish on the surface of the denture causes pain on seating the denture at a site which the patient can precisely locate. All such visible defects should have been eliminated prior to the dentures' being returned to the surgery. If, therefore, at this stage it can be felt by the patient, it cannot always be seen by the operator. A cotton wool roll drawn over the surface will reveal it by drawing out a wisp of cotton wool.

Following initial correction of any occlusal errors, pain may be felt when both dentures are in occlusion. This is probably a result of a more significant distortion of the fitting surface. The likely causes of this distortion are sites where the impression material has been penetrated by the tray, so producing distortion of the soft tissues. Alternatively the model surface (usually the crest of the ridge) might have been damaged during the technical stages.

Two materials serve to identify such defects of the fitting surface prior to their adjustment. Disclosing wax is a white wax which is melted in a suitable container and applied to the entire fitting surface using a soft brush. The tip of the brush is then used to roughen the smooth surface. After inserting the dentures and requesting the patient to close firmly, areas of excess pressure are revealed where pressure has caused the wax to be smoothed, or even extruded entirely away from the surface of the denture.

Pressure-indicating paste is a fast-setting silicone paste which is smeared over the fitting surface of the denture; then the denture is reinserted and the patient again asked to occlude firmly. Penetration of the paste by the denture base indicates points of pressure.

Lack of security

When a patient complains of an insecure denture, first diagnose whether it is a fault of retention or stability. Insecurity at rest points to a lack of retention, and, in the absence of a complaint of hyposalivation or a significant drug history, lack of peripheral seal must be suspected. Insecurity which only comes on during function (speaking and eating) is usually an indication of instability. Interference with muscle function or alternatively lack of attention to siting the teeth in the neutral zone should be suspected. Insecurity which only occurs when the patient occludes points to an occlusal error (see below). Normally the retention of an upper denture is sufficient to prevent any insecurity that may be attributable to most minor defects of stability. So poor is the retention of a lower denture, however, that even minor defects of stability can cause objectionable insecurity. As a corollary most corrections of retention relate to the upper denture and most corrections of stability to the lower denture.

When the retention of an upper denture is poor, the site of the inadequate seal must be identified. The denture is maintained in position by hand and rocked in each direction to identify the site where the seal is lacking. When displacement distally points to a lack of posterior seal, and the palatal extension of the denture is adequate, a functional post dam is placed. Autopolymerizing acrylic or chairside reline material is mixed and, when it reaches a dough consistency, is beaded over the distal edge of the tissue surface of the denture and placed into the mouth, and the patient is asked to occlude. After a few seconds the denture is removed and the set of the resin is accelerated by immersion in warm water. The addition is then smoothed and polished.

When a facial or buccal seal is required, or an underextension is to be corrected (possibly because the impression was underextended or excess acrylic was removed from the periphery at the polishing stage), additions are made to the periphery of the denture – this time with Greenstick composition. When it is felt that a seal has been re-established a wash is taken over the addition, using zinc oxide or silicone impression material, and a permanent addition is cured into place and polished carefully. Improvements to the retention of a lower denture can be made in the same way.

When instability is diagnosed it is difficult to correct the fault immediately at the chairside unless the instability is a result of overextension on to muscle insertions. Then the commonest errors are overextensions on to the mandibular and maxillary insertions of the buccinator, overextensions on to the insertion of the labial muscles, and tongue interferences with excessively long lingual extensions of lower dentures. In all cases the overextensions are identified by traction on the appropriate muscles (in the case of the tongue it is protruded) and reduction of the interfering flange.

If instability is caused by teeth not being in the neutral zone, correction is more difficult. Sometimes it is possible to remove faulty lower anterior teeth and, after a re-try, replace them in a more stable position; but it is usually easier to remake the denture. If the lack of stability can be traced to a posterior lingual undercut in the lingual polished surface of the lower denture, the fault can sometimes be cured by removing the lingual molar cusps along with the associated undercut.

Occlusal errors

Errors in the occlusion are very common, especially when the alveolar ridges are atrophic and the registration blocks insecure. Often, because the wax try-in is equally insecure, the errors remain unnoticed. Errors may occur even when the clinical stages are perfect, because the processing of a denture can introduce errors – especially if a conventional pack and press dough process is used. The pressure at the packing stage can drive individual teeth into the investing plaster to produce a premature contact, which can also occur when there is excess flash at the periphery of the flask. Occlusal errors are corrected by a precontact check record and remount, and so common are such errors that it is probably safest to perform this procedure as a routine at the insertion stage.

Technique for precontact check record

First a recording medium is placed on the posterior occlusal surfaces of the lower denture. This can be a quick-setting silicone bite registration paste, or a small amount of silicone putty mixed with excess catalyst to accelerate the set and bonded to the teeth with adhesive. Some operators get good results with softened wax, but skill is required to ensure that a similar degree of softening is achieved on both sides simultaneously. The patient is encouraged to close in the retruded contact position, but warned not to allow the artificial teeth to meet. This precaution is taken to avoid displacement of either denture as a result of cuspal interference. The patient should practise the actions to be carried out beforehand to ensure the recording is carried out without error.

When the occlusal record has set, the dentures are removed and sealed together more securely with sticky wax before being returned to the laboratory for mounting on an articulator. With no technician on the premises, the operator or a suitably trained auxiliary can carry this out. Special articulators are available for mounting dentures, using alginate as the mounting medium.

After removing the incisal pin, premature contacts are identified using thin articulating paper, and the marks of opposing cusps are deepened into fossae until even contact is achieved. Once even contact is present, smooth articulation in lateral excursions is produced by use of the BULL rule to remove interferences on each balancing side in turn. Finally the dentures are removed, cleaned of dye material, and returned to the patient.

Problems at review or later

Pain

Pain at the review stage, from either recently constructed dentures or ones made some weeks earlier, may arise from one or more of four sites:

Pain in the TMJ region
Denture-related pain at this site is usually due to lack of freeway space, but is often masked by pain from the lower denture bearing area, which tends to be more acute. The latter pain can be relieved by applying a soft liner to the fitting surface of the lower denture (which works despite the further increase in face height), but this leaves the TMJ pain unaltered.

If the dentures are some years old, pain in the TMJ region may be the result of osteo-arthritis and/or overclosure. Diagnosis may then be made when relief follows small increases in face height brought about by placing a vacuum-formed soft acrylic splint on the lower denture.

Cheek and lip biting
Cheek and lip biting are usually caused by lack of buccal or labial overjet. In the posterior region the buccal cusps of the lower teeth are reduced to increase the overjet – except when a cross-bite is present, when the buccal cusps of the upper posterior teeth are reduced. Anteriorly the process is more difficult, because the operator must keep within the bounds of good appearance. Usually there is some latitude for emphasizing the maxillary lingual incisal facets without affecting appearance, and small reductions of the labial-incisal surfaces of the lower incisors are unnoticeable if carried out with care.

Further posteriorly, nipping of the cheek mucosa can occur between the bases of the dentures in the tuberosity and retromolar pad regions, and can be relieved by thinning the bases in this region to allow a 3–4 mm gap, which should be sufficient to overcome the problem.

Sometimes cheek biting occurs when the freeway space is a little larger than the patient is accustomed to. Unless the jaw and occlusal relations are abnormal this can safely be left, and usually clears up as the patient adapts over the first few weeks.

Soreness of the tongue

If comparison with previous dentures shows that the tongue space is cramped, new dentures must be made with more space provided. In mild cases, removing the lingual cusps of the mandibular molars sometimes produces sufficient additional space.

Alternatively, the lingual surfaces of dentures might be a source of irritation to the tip of the tongue, either because they are unpolished or because there are irregularities of the teeth. Diastemas between the upper central incisors or irregularity of the lower incisors are the commoner causes. Rough surfaces are polished and irregularities smoothed. When a diastema is desired for appearance but acts as a source of irritation it can be filled with clear acrylic resin and appearance can thus be preserved.

Pain from the denture-bearing area

When dealing with pain from the denture-bearing area, first identify whether it is from the periphery or sited more centrally in the denture-bearing area.

Peripheral source of pain. Pain from the periphery of the denture-bearing area is usually associated with redness and even ulceration. The cause is extension of the denture over the insertion of the muscles at the periphery, and reduction of the base will immediately relieve the pain. The painful area can be located in relationship to the denture by first drying the mucosa, and then applying to the painful area a spot of the white zinc oxide paste component of zinc oxide impression paste. On insertion and removal of the dried denture the paste will adhere preferentially to the denture base, and thus indicate the site for reduction.

A common site for pain of this nature is in the lower posterior buccal region, just lateral to the junction of body and ramus of the mandible. This occurs because impressions are normally taken using an open-mouth technique, with the condyle displaced forwards in the glenoid fossa and the masseter muscle relaxed and displaced relatively distally. During mastication the condyle is in the retruded position in the glenoid fossa, and the masseter, now displaced forwards, contracts and crushes the mucosa and underlying buccinator muscle between itself and the disto-buccal margin of the lower denture. The contracted muscle can be palpated on occlusion, and the denture relieved in relation to it.

Central source of pain. Pain from a central area part of the denture-bearing area is more difficult to diagnose, and cases are best subdivided into those in which the pain is diffuse and associated with redness occurring over much of the denture-bearing surface, and those where it is more localized.

Diffuse source of pain. In an elderly person, if the condition is diffuse, and especially if it has occurred with previous dentures, the painful area may be a consequence of having a thin friable mucosa or of hyposalivation; the latter may be a result of drug therapy, radiotherapy or systemic disease, such as Sjögren's disease. Treatment of pain from a friable mucosa is perplexing, but sometimes it can be relieved by using a semi-permanent soft liner (e.g. Molloplast-B, Regneri GmbH, Germany). When it is caused by hyposalivation, however, silicone rubber-based semi-permanent soft liners, which tend to increase the friction between the mucosa and the denture base, make the pain worse. Instead it can be helped by prescription of an artificial saliva – Saliva Orthana (Nycomed, Birmingham, UK) is one popular, well-tolerated aerosol formulation.

When the diffuse pain began immediately after the current dentures were inserted the cause is likely to be of occlusal origin – often lack of freeway space – and the jaw and occlusal relations should be checked. When a lack of freeway space is detected, a temporary soft liner should be applied to relieve the symptoms and new dentures should be made at once. Other errors of occlusal relations can be corrected by carrying out a precontact check record. Moderate reductions of face height can also be achieved by adjustment of the occlusal surfaces in this way, but at the expense of some deterioration in appearance.

Localized source of pain. When the impression technique has been poor and the tray has penetrated the impression localized areas of the mucoperiosteum are compressed, and, when reproduced in the working model, will result in an ill-fitting painful denture. Similarly, if the model has been cast from plaster which has not been vacuum-mixed, small air bubbles beneath the surface cause a point of weakness in the plaster, and, under the packing pressure, pimples of acrylic can be produced. Both types of imperfection are identified either by sight or by use of pressure-indicating paste.

Alternatively, a localized painful area associated with inflammation can occur either when an unnoticed undercut in the denture abrades the soft tissues – usually over a prominence of the alveolus or the mylohyoid ridge, or when there is pressure on a prominent midline or mandibular torus. The pain is removed by reduction of the denture base in the appropriate area.

Discrete painful areas without any associated inflammation may occur in two areas, viz over a superficial mental nerve or over sharp bony spicules where resorption has been irregular – usually in the lower anterior region. Radiographs reveal the cause (sharp bony spicules may require a radiograph with reduced exposure). Pain over the mental foramen is relieved by reducing the denture base in relation to the foramen. Treatment of irregular resorption is a surgical problem. If surgery is contra-indicated, as with many elderly people, provision of a semi-permanent soft lining can sometimes be helpful, but can often make things much worse, especially if there is a degree of hyposalivation.

Sometimes inspection of the painful area reveals it to be associated with a sinus, when an underlying root or other pathology must be suspected. If this is confirmed by radiograph it must be removed.

Lack of denture security

In general the diagnosis and treatment of lack of security at this stage is the same as at the insertion stage. Additional causes of denture insecurity specific to this stage are interference with the modiolus or the coronoid process, lack of tolerance, cuspal interference, and other occlusal faults.

Interference with the modiolus

Unless the modiolus is supported by the upper premolar teeth, it can act to displace the lower denture. If the lower premolar teeth are buccally displaced, usually in the presence of a Class III jaw relationship, their buccal cusps must be reduced.

Interference with the coronoid process

On rare occasions the upper denture may be destabilized when opening the mouth owing to contact between the coronoid process and an excessively thick posterior maxillary buccal flange. Thinning the buccal flange in this region is usually sufficient.

Lack of tolerance
An elderly person may take a considerable time to adapt to the shape of a new denture, and may complain of insecurity despite a great increase in retention. If adaptation does not occur, replacement of the denture by one which is a copy of the original usually cures the problem.

Cuspal interference
When a patient has become used to an occlusal form which is flat as a consequence of attrition and abrasion, replacement by a denture with anatomical cusp forms can result in instability. By remounting on an articulator the occlusal surface can be adjusted and the cusps reduced in height while occlusal balance is maintained.

Other occlusal faults
Sometimes the occlusal relations of a denture which is due for replacement are far from normal. Freeway spaces which are judged to be normal at the insertion stage may be insufficient when the original freeway space was excessive, and unless the patient's potential for tolerating change has been investigated by incremental change to the old occlusal surfaces, new dentures with apparently normal freeway space can cause instability. A reduction of the face height on an articulator via a remount can be carried out, and sometimes a satisfactory result is achieved.

Rarely, provision of the appearance that the patient asks for might lead to an occlusal plane which is higher than the maximum convexity of the tongue. The lower denture may then be unstable.

Inability to chew

Complaints of inability to chew are usually due to occlusal problems, either lack of freeway space or a premature contact. If possible, correction is carried out on an articulator after recording the occlusal relations with a check record. Rarely the inability to chew is caused by restriction of the tongue space. Treatment then involves replacement of the dentures with a view to an increase of the available tongue space.

When the complaint of inability to chew arises after some years of normal service, the cause is usually an increase in freeway space along with an associated loss of the anatomical shape of the tooth cusps. While the patient is more aware of the latter of these changes, the former must not be overlooked.

Numbness of the lip

With atrophy of the mandibular alveolus the mental foramen approaches the crest of the residual ridge, and may become part of the lower denture-bearing area. Pressure from the lower denture can then cause numbness of the lower lip in the distribution of the mental nerve. Relief of the denture base in the region of the mental foramen is necessary. Application of a semi-permanent soft lining tends only to make the situation worse.

Interference with speech

Two types of fault commonly cause interference with speech following provision of new dentures. Lack of freeway space causes sibilance of speech or even a frank complaint that speech is difficult or altered. This complaint is therefore useful to confirm the diagnosis of a freeway space problem. When the speech complaint is not associated with pain from the lower denture-bearing area – for example, when it is part of a plan to reduce an excessive loss of face height – gradual adaptation occurs, but more quickly with young patients.

Interference with labio-dental and linguo-dental sounds ('f' and 'th') is the result of incorrect placement of the upper anterior teeth, or the correct placement of upper anterior teeth for a patient who has had them incorrectly placed for some time. Again, adaptation will occur swiftly in a relatively young patient, but in a longer time for a patient with diminished powers of adaptation. Where the molars are set in an arch which is wider than that to which the patient is accustomed, some linguo-palatal sounds ('cl') are converted to a 'shushing' sound. Again, adaptation will occur after reassurance.

Other types of denture

Patients with partial dentures or overdentures can also present with complaints which require immediate attention. Most are analogous to those of complete dentures and can be treated in the same way. Some are specific, especially those relating to implant-retained overdentures, and their treatment warrants separate discussion.

Partial dentures

Complaints due to complete overbite or nausea

It is difficult to design a conventional temporary partial denture for a patient with a complete overbite. Either the base fractures repeatedly or the lower anterior teeth must be reduced far enough to permit passage of an acrylic connector of adequate thickness. A temporary alternative to the conventional design is to make a labial veneer denture. This is retained by means of a thin acrylic veneer which passes over the buccal surface of the alveolus back to the premolar teeth, obtaining its retention by entering the small interproximal undercuts posteriorly. Palatal support is limited, and passes only as far posteriorly as the point of contact between the lower anterior teeth and the palate. The denture will act as a temporary replacement for missing anterior teeth, and if used as an immediate appliance can be lined with soft lining material to restore fit as resorption occurs. Because the denture has minimal support from tissues capable of resisting masticatory stresses, it is provided principally to restore appearance, but can be used for function if care is taken. The same difficulty arises when the partial denture designed to temporarily replace a missing anterior tooth gives rise to nausea, and is solved in the same way.

Fracture of the denture

Fracture of an acrylic-base partial denture is common. Acrylic-base dentures are rarely adequately supported by teeth, and instead rely on support by the soft tissues. The change in shape of the soft tissue support which follows alveolar resorption soon produces a discrepancy between the denture and its supporting tissues, and the resulting stress concentration can cause fracture. It is rarely worthwhile repairing such fractures except on a temporary basis. Repair with inclusion of a strengthening material which has no adhesive bond with the acrylic base merely increases the likelihood of another fracture. Temporary repairs can be made as for complete dentures provided the pieces can be reapposed accurately out of the mouth. If this is impossible, an impression can be taken in alginate with the denture in the mouth and a model cast containing the denture. A repair is carried out in the normal way.

Fracture of metal base components is not uncommon, provided that there are no inclusions of air or foreign material in the casting. Following such a fracture the denture may be unwearable, and a new one should be made as quickly as possible. Fracture of a cast metal clasp is the commonest finding, especially if the clasp has required adjustment at the insertion stage or if the metal has been thinned to allow for occlusal interferences. Some loss of retention follows, but the denture may still function, and the presenting symptom is irritation from the sharp metal. The sharp ends should be smoothed with a carborundum disc before being polished with rubber wheels. If it is decided that retention must be improved in the short term, then provided that there is a suitable adjacent site of attachment, a wrought stainless steel clasp can be added. An impression is first taken in alginate with the denture in the patient's mouth. The clasp is then added on the model.

Caries of an abutment tooth

The presence of a partial denture exacts from the patient a biological price in terms of a diminution in oral health and increased proneness to plaque accumulation and susceptibility to caries and periodontal disease. Despite careful assessment and encouragement of adequate oral hygiene habits, caries of abutment teeth can occur. If the caries is at the cervical margin or surfaces which do not contact the denture, a conventional restoration is carried out. When the caries involves replacement of a restoration containing a rest seat it is often best to replace the defective restoration with an inlay. An overcontoured pattern is prepared directly in the mouth. The contacting denture surface is Vaselined, warmed and placed into position. Surplus inlay wax is carved down and the direct pattern removed, sprued and cast. After checking that good functional contact occurs between the partial denture and the inlay, it is cemented into place under occlusal pressure with the denture in the mouth. Direct composite inlays can be made in an analogous way.

When a larger restoration is required, namely one which involves more than three surfaces, it is best to provide a crown. After making the preparation and taking impressions, a die is cast on which the technician prepares an autopolymerizing acrylic resin core. The core is placed in the mouth and waxed up directly into a crown. The warmed denture coated with separating medium is inserted at intervals to avoid overcontouring. A similar procedure is carried out if a crown on an abutment tooth requires replacement.

Loss of a natural tooth

Loss of a natural posterior tooth does not often demand its immediate addition to a partial denture, but loss of an anterior tooth is much more urgent. Provided that there is an adjacent part of the denture to which attachment can be gained there are no special difficulties. Addition to an acrylic-base partial denture requires no more than an impression with the denture in the patient's mouth and an appropriate shade. With care and cleanliness a good bond can be produced between the added tooth and the denture base. A cast metal base is more difficult to add to, and mechanical dovetails must be cut into the metal into which the addition can lock. If this is impossible owing to the shape of the base (for example, the adjacent metal may be too thin to give three-dimensional interlocking) or because the adjacent metal is a lingual bar connector, an accessory bonding system is used. Bonding the addition to the metal base with 4 META resin is the treatment of choice, and it may be advisable to use this form of bonding in all cases when acrylic to metal attachment is required.

Loss of a tooth from the denture

Loss of a tooth from the denture implies that the original bonding was deficient, or was insufficient to withstand unanticipated stresses. The denture tooth can be reattached. Again, it is best to use a 4 META resin in all cases where acrylic to metal bonding is needed.

Conventional overdentures

Insecurity due to lack of functional support

When preparing a temporary or transitional overdenture the base is processed on a model which is trimmed to represent the final situation which will be produced clinically when the overdenture abutments are reduced. To ensure that interferences are not produced the future abutment teeth on the model are reduced to about 1 mm higher than the preferred final height. Following the actual reduction in the mouth a space will now exist between the base and the abutment surfaces. To restore functional contact a small amount of autopolymerizing acrylic is placed on the denture base at the abutment site. After Vaselining the abutments the denture is placed into the mouth and held under occlusal pressure until the acrylic has set. The denture is then removed and excess acrylic trimmed away. Some clinicians advise that when preparing a permanent overdenture a small space should be allowed between the denture base and the abutment surfaces so that stresses are only applied to the teeth during function. To permit this, foil may be placed over the abutments before processing the acrylic denture base, or if a metal denture base is to be made, before laying down the wax pattern.

Although the majority of overdenture abutments remain with the occlusal surface of the root face restored merely by a glass–ionomer or composite resin, some clinicians advise that as a final restoration cast metal diaphragms should be provided. Such restorations do not inhibit or prevent caries in any way, and can only serve either to provide better security by allowing a more dome-shaped preparation or to reduce wear of the abutment when it is in contact with a metal base. They should only be provided when a permanent overdenture is being made and a clear need for this form of restoration has been established.

Caries

Caries of the exposed dentine surface is a very common cause of overdenture failure, and patients must be warned of this possible consequence. Unless patients who request overdenture therapy are carefully selected and their caries rates are assessed and their role in the maintenance of oral hygiene is emphasized, caries of the abutments will be inevitable. Aids to oral hygiene must include use of a fluoridated toothpaste, not only for removing plaque but for applying in small quantities as a topical agent to the fitting surface of the denture in contact with the abutments. Fluoridated mouthrinses should be advised, and, at review, fluoride varnishes can be applied to the exposed abutment surfaces.

Base fracture

Fracture of acrylic-based overdentures is common owing to the decreased bulk of the denture where the abutments protrude into the denture space. To prevent fracture of a permanent overdenture a cast metal base can be provided. This need not cover the labial surface of the ridge (where it might affect appearance) but can be confined to the lingual side, passing forwards to the crest of the ridge. If required, functional spacing between the base and the abutment teeth can be achieved by placing foil of the desired thickness on the model before laying down the pattern.

Implant-supported overdentures

Although implant placement is associated with a high degree of success, no appliance placed in the mouth is immune to problems. Now that implant-retained overdentures are a popular form of prosthesis for the atrophic edentulous mandible, even practitioners who do not provide this form of treatment must be aware of the problems that can arise and be prepared to treat them if they are to give a comprehensive service to their patients.

Soft tissue infection

Soft tissue infections in relation to an implant fixture are uncommon, and although no definite associations have been made with lack of oral hygiene, it is the impression of many that they are commoner when oral hygiene is neglected or when the permucosal part of the implant is not surrounded by attached mucoperiosteum.

On examination the soft tissues around the implant are swollen and the regional lymph nodes may be enlarged and tender. The associated pain may prevent the patient wearing the denture. Because the infection involves only the soft tissues, integration is unaffected and the fixture is firm and painless to percussion. Radiographic examination shows no bony changes. Testing with a Periotest, if available, is a useful supplementary means of diagnosis and integration is confirmed when it gives a reading of between −5 and +5, indicating that integration is equivalent to that of an ankylosed root.

Treatment involves thorough prophylaxis of the gingival crevice and removal of deposits from the implant surface. Prescription of antibiotics is not usually indicated, although slow-release tetracycline and metronidazole, as used in periodontal therapy, may be installed in the gingival crevice. The patient is encouraged to practise vigorous oral hygiene measures. When the infection resolves, the denture can be worn once more. Recurrence of the infection is an indication for flap surgery in order to ensure that the fixture is surrounded by firm, attached mucoperiosteum.

Loss of integration

At review a patient may complain that there is pain on chewing, and loss of integration of a fixture may be suspected. On examination the affected fixture will be tender to percussion, and the Periotest reading greater than +5. Radiographs showing bone loss in relation to the fixture confirm the diagnosis. If the fixture is relatively firm the overdenture can be removed, the transmucosal part of the implant removed under local analgesia, a sealing screw placed and the perforation in the mucosa allowed to heal.

Later, if another unused adjacent fixture is available, a new overdenture can be made involving it. This procedure is relatively simple if the overdenture is one which is retained by studs, when the remaining stud permits adequate, if reduced, retention. Where a Dolder bar or milled bar type of attachment is involved, the bar must be entirely removed, a procedure which compromises the security of the denture until a new one can be made.

Where no other fixtures are available an attempt can be made to reintegrate the affected fixture by leaving it buried for a further period of at least 3 months in the mandible and 6 months in the maxilla. Again, the procedure is much easier when stud retention has been employed.

Sometimes loss of integration is so great that during attempts to remove the transmucosal part, the fixture is found to move freely. Under these circumstances the fixture is removed and appropriate adjustments are made to the overdenture. Later, when healing has occurred, a new fixture can be placed, in either the same or an adjacent site.

Loose stud element

In the case of overdentures retained by studs, the stud screws directly into the fixture using either a hex or a conventional driver. Ideally this should be inserted by means of an electrical torque-control device, when the recommended torques are easier to apply without slipping. When driven by hand the studs may not be tightened adequately – especially when the design of the stud demands a conventional rather than a hex driver.

When a patient reports one of his or her implants becoming loose and loosening of the stud element is suspected the patient must attend the surgery immediately. If this is impossible patients must be advised that if the stud element is merely loose and not completely detached they should attempt to screw it back in by hand (but never by using a mechanical device). When, later, the patient attends the surgery the stud can be re-tightened adequately. Should the stud become completely detached from the fixture the access hole through the mucosa will close quickly, and it rapidly becomes impossible to replace the stud without damaging or trapping the soft tissues. Under these circumstances a flap is raised and the site of the fixture is exposed surgically before the stud is replaced. The same stipulation applies if there is pain when the stud is tightened. Soft tissues are almost certainly being trapped between the stud and fixture. Surgical exposure of the site is mandatory, and the stud is placed under direct vision.

Silicone-based adhesives are available to improve the bond between a fixture and the retaining screw. However, their usefulness is limited. For maximum effect they must be applied to dry surfaces. Without exposing the site surgically it is exceedingly difficult to keep the screw thread of a fixture (especially a mandibular fixture) dry for more than a few seconds. In addition, the adhesive fills in the gap between the threads of the fixture and the retaining screw, a gap which some manufacturers deliberately leave in order to prevent pressure build-up in the fixture cavity.

Insecurity of the overdenture

When patients complain of a loose overdenture careful investigation will show the cause to be either lack of support of the distal saddle of the denture due to alveolar resorption, or wear of the attachment itself.

Lack of support

Alveolar resorption beneath the distal extension of an implant-supported overdenture leads to the complaint of movement of the denture. Examination of the denture in the mouth reveals that, with the retentive devices fully engaged, the distal extension can be further displaced towards the ridge. Relining of the denture will correct this fault.

Relining an implant-supported overdenture is analogous to relining a conventional denture, and any undercuts are first removed. The reline impression is then taken in a medium-bodied silicone impression paste, with the dentures in light occlusion. On removal from the mouth any excess impression material which has extended beyond the fitting surface is excised. After blocking out the retentive mechanism, a model is cast. The denture is invested as normal and relined in heat-cured acrylic.

Wear of attachment

When an overdenture is retained by a Dolder bar the constant movement of the denture causes wear of the retaining elements. To some extent this can be compensated for by adjustment of the spring. Ultimately this becomes no longer possible, and a new overdenture must be made.

In the same way wear and loss of retention of stud attachments occurs. When the female element is a metal spring cup held in tension by a silicone washer, replacement of the silicone washer is indicated, and is a relatively simple procedure. It can be performed by either the operator or a technician using the appropriate tools. Other forms of stud retainer depend for all their retention on a silicone ring encircling the titanium stud. In these cases the silicone ring is normally replaced every year or so, and spares are supplied with the kit.

When loss of retention has occurred to such an extent that replacement of the entire female part of the retainer is warranted, the device is replaced by means of a local addition using autopolymerizing resin. The worn part is cut from the denture and a new cup and/or retaining silicone washer are placed in position on the male element. Any undercuts in the assembly on the male element are then blocked out with soft wax. After ensuring that the denture fits over the new stud without interference, a mix of autopolymerizing resin is made and used to anchor the female part of the new stud to the denture.

Because repair and additions to stud attachments are so much easier than to bar attachments there is a tendency for bar devices to be converted to stud attachments when they become worn. Conversion kits can be purchased to allow this, and first involve removing the bar and replacing the transmucosal element with an appropriate stud. The two parts of the retaining device are located either directly, as above, or indirectly in the laboratory.

4

Endodontics

Philip Wragg

Introduction

The potential for problems in endodontics is great, and is increased by the fact that the majority of instrumentation is done 'blind', albeit assisted by radiographs to estimate the length of root canals. Hence an intimate knowledge of root canal morphology is the first requisite for good practice. Fortunately, despite the many potential difficulties, and the complexity of the procedures, it is unusual for a tooth to give rise to problems, despite even poorly executed procedures. When things do go wrong, it is important that the dentist recognizes the problem and, more importantly, knows how to deal with it appropriately. This may involve treatment by the dental practitioner, or in some cases, referral to a person with specialist knowledge and skills for advice, and/or treatment.

Whilst the following chapter is by no means an authoritative guide to the full range of endodontic difficulties that the dental practitioner might encounter in his or her practice, it does consider some of the more common problems and give an insight into cause, treatment, and avoidance; although this last can by no means be guaranteed.

Difficult penetration of the canal

The tooth which has been treated endodontically presents many problems, even to an experienced operator. Common complaints are that the root canal is difficult to find, difficult to negotiate, or blocked by some internal obstruction or earlier form of endodontic therapy. In many instances the problems can be overcome with the exercise of sufficient care.

Canals which are difficult to find or negotiate

There are many reasons why a root canal may prove difficult to find. If we ignore operator variables such as clinical experience and knowledge of root canal morphology (and variations), the usual causes are either sclerosis or obliteration, or deceptive angulation of the crown.

Sclerosis or obliteration of the canal

Sclerosis or obliteration of the root canal is sometimes seen in teeth which have been traumatized, and may on occasion be so extensive that there is no evidence of a canal on radiograph. If this is the case, it is possible that a conventional orthograde approach to treatment will be unsuccessful, and consideration should be given to recommending alternative forms of treatment. These might include apical surgery or extraction.

Where sclerosis of the root canal is due to age changes it is often less complete. In such a situation, secondary dentine may make a conventional approach difficult, but not necessarily impossible. Whilst such canals may prove difficult to locate or penetrate, they should be amenable to treatment as long as the canal, though very fine, is detectable on the radiograph.

Often, the only clinical evidence of canal presence is a change in colour due to secondary dentine formation, which has tended to obliterate the canal. This is usually darker than the surrounding dentine, giving a visual clue to the whereabouts of the canal. In this situation, careful exploration and preparation are required. A fine endodontic explorer such as the EXDG16 (Hu-Friedy, Chicago, Illinois, US) is helpful for locating the entrance to root canals. Whilst not essential, visual magnification by loupes is desirable (the choice is a matter of personal preference).

Once identified, the entrance to the canal may be carefully enlarged by means of Gates–Glidden burs. Burs of this type have a long shank and come in a range of sizes (1–6). Designed with a non-cutting tip, they are used incrementally to enlarge the openings of root canals and refine the canal shape (flare) in the coronal two-thirds. Judicious use early in preparation will facilitate the passage of instruments to the working length, and ultimately promote satisfactory obturation.

Copious irrigation should be used at all times to reduce the chances of instruments' binding and minimize the build-up of debris in the canal. In some instances chelating agents and similar products may be used according to the manufacturers' instruction. More often these products are used for their lubricating properties.

Deceptive angulation

A pre-operative radiograph is essential for adequate diagnosis. Not only does it yield information about the root canal and root morphology, but it can also reveal any deviation of the root canal from the crown. Nowhere is this more important than in a tooth which has been crowned. Many tipped or rotated teeth are crowned so as to disguise the situation that existed before treatment, and this can mask the true orientation of the crown to the root. All too often the dentist will press on in his search for the canal without an adequate preliminary radiograph, and it is in this way that many root canals are inadvertently perforated. In such cases it is often better to remove the crown to assess the true angulation. This in turn facilitates preparation of the access cavity and ensures that the preparation remains within the long axis of the root. In summary, it is best to be cautious, particularly where the crown was placed by another dentist.

Obstruction of the canal by an instrument or post

Obstruction of the canal is a common problem. Whether it is a result of misadventure during treatment, an incidental finding on radiograph, or the result of earlier conventional endodontic treatment, is to some extent irrelevant; what is important is that it may preclude further endodontic therapy or compromise the long-term prognosis of the tooth. Where the problem can not be overcome, alternative approaches or possible extraction may be required. The two common reasons for canal obstruction are broken instruments and fractured posts or dowels.

Broken instruments

For ease of discussion, and because each has its own technique for removal, broken instruments can be considered under the categories of hand- or engine-driven types.

Hand instruments

Modern hand instruments, such as endodontic files, spreaders and explorers, rarely break in use. When they do so, it is usually a result of misuse or abuse. Take for example endodontic files. These instruments are, on the whole, designed for use with a filing action. When used with a rotational action, there is a risk of the instrument's wedging. If this happens, the machined portion of the file may be twisted and strained, resulting in permanent deformation.

Continuing to turn the instrument in such circumstances is likely to result in the fatigue strength of the instrument being exceeded, and possible fracture. Even if the instrument does not break, there is the danger that the damage may not be noticed, so that an 'inexplicable' break occurs at the next use. For these reasons, any rotary action should be limited to a maximum of one quarter turn, particularly in small sizes (<No. 35), where the risks of deformation and breakage are so much greater. Instruments below size 35 are best regarded as being for one-time use only and discarded after each patient. All instruments should be examined visually before use, and discarded if there are obvious signs of damage.

Even with new instruments, there is always a small risk of breakage. This can be minimized by avoiding their use in a dry canal, when not only is there a danger of the canal becoming clogged with debris, but also the risk of wedging and fracturing the instrument owing to the lack of a lubricant effect. A suitable irrigant is sodium hypochlorite in a concentration of between 0.5 per cent and 5.25 per cent. If an instrument does become tight in use, return to a smaller size (recapitulation) before trying the next larger size. Not only will this minimize the opportunity for wedging of an instrument, but it will also reduce the chances of the canal becoming blocked with debris apically.

To summarize, in order to reduce the likelihood of fracture of hand instruments:

- Never reuse small instruments (<No. 35).
- Never rotate beyond one quarter turn.
- Always lubricate canals; never use instruments in dry canals.
- Always inspect instruments before and regularly during use.
- Never force instruments; always return to a smaller size if an instrument becomes tight during use.

Engine-driven instruments

Rotary instruments, such as Gates–Glidden burs, Peso reamers and twist drills, are commonly used during the preparation of the canal to receive a dowel or post. Spiral fillers are often used to fill the canal with sealant. Of the above, the spiral filler is, perhaps, the most abused and frequently broken instrument. As a precaution, when using spiral fillers, they should be cut two to three millimetres short of the working length, and a size should be used that freely rotates within the canal. This will greatly reduce the risk of breakage.

Whilst the larger sizes of any engine-driven instrument will resist misuse by even the most determined operator, the smaller sizes may occasionally break during use, particularly if lateral forces are applied, as might be the case when used in a curved canal. This might also happen when attempts are made to free an instrument wedged in the canal. In the event of an instrument wedging, try reversing the motor. If this fails, detach the instrument from the chuck of the handpiece. This allows application of controlled force, by grasping the instrument in Spencer Wells forceps or a similar device. Rotation in an anti-clockwise direction will usually free the instrument. In order to minimize further the risk of wedging and provide greater control, use the instrument in a speed-reducing handpiece at moderate speed together with an irrigant. This will be beneficial, the irrigant acting as a cooling medium and lubricant, in addition to carrying away debris.

Finally, unless there is straight-line access to the root canal, and these instruments are used only in the straight portion of the canal, there is the risk of the instrument being diverted off course, with consequent perforation.

Therefore, for successful endodontics and to minimize the risk of failure through instrument breakage:

- Take care when using in canals with a curve (toward the apex).
- Never force or allow instruments to wedge or become jammed.
- Always ensure adequate and straight-line access.
- Always use a lubricant.
- Never re-use small instruments.
- Always discard instruments which are bent or appear damaged.

Dealing with the broken instrument

If you are lucky, the instrument will be accessible to a pair of fine mosquito or similar forceps. If you are unlucky, the fragment will be out of direct grasp by such an approach; then, in the case of fine endodontic instruments, whether the instrument can be removed depends upon how much force was put into wedging it there. Sometimes it is possible to take one or two endodontic files, and after wrapping them around the fragment, retrieve it.

The Masserann kit was developed by Jean Masserann (distributed and produced by Micro-Méga, France), and consists of a series of hollow trephines. Although generally used for the retrieval of broken posts (see Chapter 2), it does contain extractors (which are available in two diameters, 1.2 mm and 1.5 mm, each having an internal locking device) that are designed to pass over the end of the broken fragment and retrieve it after securing it within the tube. This is not always successful, and depends on the canal being of adequate diameter, or capable of being enlarged to allow free passage of the extractor.

Where the fragment proves impossible to remove, it may be possible to prepare and fill the canal leaving the instrument in situ, entombing it with the final obturation of the canal. If this has to be done, warn the patient. If the patient is not warned there may be the risk of litigation at some future date.

Finally, in a difficult case, it is always worth telephoning the local dental hospital or the nearest consultant in restorative dentistry, who would usually be only too pleased to help.

Obstruction of the canal by an earlier root filling

A canal which has been instrumented to create an apical stop from where the canal gently flares coronally to the access cavity, and is then obturated with gutta percha and a sealant such as Grossman's sealer, will present no problem in the event that re-treatment is required. Gutta percha is a material which can easily be softened by the application of heat or solvent, or removed by the use of Gates–Glidden burs or their equivalents.

The problem arises where gutta percha has not been used or, for example, where a rigid-setting sealer has been used. It can then be very difficult to remove the sealer without the risk of damage to the canal or root perforation. Although the technique is now outdated, perhaps the greatest difficulty is caused where silver points have been used to obturate the canal. This is a technique which enjoyed wide application, especially for narrow canals. It required the canal to be 'reamed' so as to provide an apical portion which was round in cross section, and relied on the presence of cement to obturate the irregularities of the canal. We now know that it is virtually impossible to create such a uniformly round and smooth shape. Modern techniques now aim for a three-dimensional fill of the canal system, which despite mechanical preparation is rarely round. Silver points not only fail to fill the canal; with time they corrode. The corrosion products may result in discoloration of the dentine and additionally weaken the silver point to the extent that if attempts are made to remove them they often break up. At least for the time being, there will remain a group of patients in whom silver points were used in the past, and, in this group, their removal and re-treatment will remain problematic.

Obstruction by an earlier post/core crown

Another area where there is often difficulty is in the re-treatment of the tooth which is already post-crowned. The decision as to whether the post should be removed to allow repeat endodontic therapy is difficult. As a rule, where the post is short or of small diameter its removal should be considered, because to leave it risks failure at some future date. In the event that the post is long and of appropriate diameter and the root is thin it is best to leave the post/core in situ rather than risk fracturing the root. Equally, where the root filling appears of adequate length and to be well condensed there may be little point in considering conventional re-treatment, and surgical treatment should be considered. In all situations, clinical judgment should prevail; but remember to assess all options and then exclude the inappropriate.

In the event that the post requires removal, there are various techniques available, and it is a question of using the most appropriate in the given circumstances. For example, if the post is of a threaded design, it may be possible carefully to unscrew it. However, check if there is an anti-rotation device. This may sometimes take the form of a small cavity at the base of the post engaging it, and the root face, and then filled with amalgam or composite or glass–ionomer cement. This should be removed first by drilling.

A cemented post can often be loosened by careful application of force through an excavator or a pair of mosquito forceps. Sometimes a proprietary post extractor can be used; but these first require the removal of the crown, and are useful mainly with upper anterior teeth. The technique of vibration of the post with an ultrasonic instrument to try to break the cement seal may also be tried; but this will often be less successful.

Finally, if removal of the post seems inappropriate and yet further endodontic intervention seems necessary, it may be that a retrograde approach is required, or, in extreme cases, extraction.

Post-operative pain

Usually pain indicates that the canal was not adequately instrumented, or that contaminated material remains or was pushed through the apex into the periapical tissues. To overcome this problem the canal must be re-instrumented adequately and all contaminated material must be removed. Sometimes pain is a sign that the temporary coronal seal has leaked, allowing contamination of the cleaned root canal system. Then the problem is overcome by placing a seal with adhesive qualities, for example a polycarboxylate cement or a glass–ionomer (polyalkenoate) cement. Occasionally, pain is a sign that there is an occlusal prematurity through overbuilding the temporary restoration; and this must always be checked after removal of the rubber dam.

Instrumentation criteria

To ensure adequate instrumentation the first requirement is good isolation. If the tooth has a cavity with margins which make isolation difficult, it must first be restored with amalgam, composite or glass–ionomer cement. Although this may be a temporary measure, and the definitive restoration may require its removal, the advantages gained in permitting effective isolation justify its use. Not only does this prevent further contamination of the root canal during preparation, but it also allows for the use of intra-canal irrigation with sodium hypochlorite, itself a powerful antibacterial agent which reduces the amount of microbiological contamination.

To reduce the amount of contaminated material further, modern teaching in endodontics suggests that canals should be instrumented using a 'crown-down' approach, rather than the standard 'step back' technique. In contrast to the latter the crown-down approach first requires instrumentation, and hence gross debridement, of the coronal two-thirds of the root canal, both by hand files and Gates–Glidden burs. This has the effect of removing the bulk of the contaminated material, so that, when it is necessary to re-take the working length radiograph and subsequently instrument the apical third, the bacterial load has been significantly reduced. Additionally, it allows unrestricted passage of files into the canal and reduces their chances of binding coronally, so facilitating obturation. The flared preparation that results also aids passage of irrigant toward the apex, further preventing the build-up of debris and reducing the chance of debris being extruded from the apex.

Even with a careful technique, there is a tendency for the debris of canal preparation to be forced through the apical foramen. This can be demonstrated by instrumenting an extracted tooth in the hand. Debris is seen to be extruded from the apical foramen like toothpaste from a tube. This inoculation of the periapical tissues with non-vital and perhaps infected tissue will often result in a rapid host response, with pain and possible abscess formation. The problem of pain from this source is difficult to deal with, and every effort must be made to prevent its occurrence. Re-capitulation, i.e. the technique whereby, after use of a file, the file a size smaller is reinserted to the working length so as to remove the build-up of debris, is essential. Copious quantities of irrigant are also recommended. Sodium hypochlorite in a concentration of between 0.5 per cent and 5.25 per cent is generally used for such a purpose.

Use of intra-canal medicaments

Modern endodontic techniques aim to prepare a root canal which has smooth walls and a gentle flare from apex to crown, free of irregularities. If they are undertaken carefully, all necrotic debris should have been removed, assisted by the flushing action of the sodium hypochlorite solution. Evidence suggests that these techniques will, if combined with use of an inert sealant, result in successful endodontic therapy.

As a rule, intra-canal medicaments or dressings have nothing further to offer in terms of success. There is, however, one exception: namely, calcium hydroxide. This material is particularly useful where a canal is persistently difficult to settle – for example, the canal that remains wet despite careful application of appropriate techniques, or the canal which has a perforation, or an 'open' apex with bleeding that has proved difficult to control. In these situations, dressing the canal with calcium hydroxide for a period of a few weeks is often of benefit.

Calcium hydroxide and barium sulphate in equal proportions mixed to a paste with sterile water are transported to the canal on a suitable instrument and packed into the canal with paper points. Gradually the canal is filled in this way, and a check radiograph is taken to confirm the fill. As an alternative, but with extreme care, a spiral canal filler may be used. Note carefully that the spiral filler should always be shortened so that it remains 2–3 mm short of the apical stop. You should also ensure that it is free to turn within the canal without binding, or else there is a risk of fracture of the instrument within the canal and compromise of an otherwise successful result. After a 'healing' interval, in which the dressing may have to be replaced periodically, the calcium hydroxide may be rinsed out of the canal and the canal dried prior to definitive obturation.

Prolonged treatment

The idea that the fill of the canal was most important has now given way to the realization that it is the preparation of the canal which is perhaps the single most important aspect of treatment. In preparing the canal to receive the final fill there are a number of aims and objectives:

- the removal of pulp remnants
- the removal of necrotic or infected material from the walls of the canal
- the creation of a smooth tapering canal, the shape of which is appropriate for the technique and material to be used for obturation.

When things do not go to plan, it is usually because the above objectives have not been met. The tooth fails to settle or flares up each time it is temporarily sealed; having to leave the tooth on open drainage is not uncommon. The most common cause of such problems, and hence of prolonged treatment, is poor access. The creation of adequate access is the key to endodontics, and its preparation in both single- and multi-rooted teeth merits two separate discussions.

Single-rooted tooth

Often when the access is examined on a troublesome anterior tooth it is seen to be circular, and often not much larger in diameter than the bur used to make it. The problem lies here. Such an access denies proper entry to the canal, and prevents removal of contents which may be necrotic or infected. Important areas to consider are the pulp horns to the mesial and distal faces in incisor teeth and the area under the cusp tips in pre-molar teeth. The access cavity should be large enough to gain unimpeded straight-line access to the canal system, including pulp horns and any irregularities. The walls of the opening should flow smoothly into the canal proper, without ledges or undercuts. When the opening is adequately prepared, it should be possible to insert an instrument without its touching the walls of the access cavity at any point. Failure to remove all debris from the tooth may result in long-term discoloration and patient dissatisfaction.

Tapered-fissure diamond burs are used to create the desired access. Preferably they should be non end-cutting, to prevent undue damage to the canal, and, in posterior teeth, the floor of the pulp chamber. Having entered the root canal, Gates–Glidden burs are used to refine the access until the preparation flows smoothly from coronal access to canal. This may be checked by use of an explorer or file, which should pass into the canal without catching.

In some teeth, particularly upper and lower anterior teeth, it is difficult to get straight-line access. It is then sometimes necessary to sacrifice some labial enamel to facilitate access. When this is necessary the reason why it is should be explained to the patient. Such damage is often acceptable, especially if a crown or veneer is to be used to restore the root-treated tooth.

Use of an irrigant is important for proper cleaning of the canal system. Sodium hypochlorite in a concentration of between 0.5 per cent and 5.25 per cent is the agent of choice. In addition to being a bleaching agent and acting as a lubricant, this can liquefy pulpal remnants and is bactericidal. It also acts as a flushing agent and, if used with a recapitulation technique, prevents build-up of debris at the apex. Because it can damage tissues it must be used with rubber dam isolation to prevent leakage, and also demands a tight marginal seal of the temporary restoration. The tip of the needle used for irrigation should pass to within a few millimetres of the apex, and must be of 25 gauge or finer, so that it does not bind on insertion; otherwise there is a risk of solution being forced through the apex.

Multi-rooted teeth

An occasional mistake when treating multi-rooted teeth is to prepare the access and believe you are in the pulp chamber, mistaking the pulp horns for the root canals, when in reality the roof of the pulp chamber is still intact. When treating a multi-rooted tooth in which access is proving difficult you should always ask yourself whether you are through the roof and into the pulp chamber proper. If the entrances to all canals are visible in your mirror, if the base of the cavity is slightly darker than the surrounding dentine, and if it is possible to see the developmental grooves which run from one orifice to another, then you probably have an adequate access. As with an anterior tooth, unimpeded, straight-line access is all-important to success. Therefore make sure the access is smooth and flowing, with no steps, ledges or irregularities to prevent entry to the canals.

Apical trauma and perforation

Unplanned trauma as a result of canal preparation during endodontic procedures may take the form of a zip, ledge or transportation, or a perforation or laceration.

Zip, ledge formation, and transportation

Zipping is a term which describes the damage done to the apical stop resulting from the tip of the instrument cutting laterally into the dentine at the apex, producing an apical stop which is no longer of circular cross section. It occurs because, when introduced into a curved canal, straight instruments have a tendency to cut at the inner aspect of the curve at the midpoint of the instrument, and at the outer aspect of the root apex at the tip. If the instrument has not been introduced as far as the apex, a 'zip' is produced more coronally. This formation is termed a ledge, and its shape and site make further penetration by an instrument towards the apex difficult. Once a zip or ledge is established, proper debridement and subsequent obturation is usually incomplete, and further instrumentation may be denied.

Transportation is the term given to the effect of filing a canal in such a way that more tooth substance is selectively removed from one wall of the canal than the other, resulting in transportation or apparent displacement of the canal when viewed in a cross section. Commonly the inner aspect of a curved canal is affected in this way, and the canal is repositioned in the direction of the inner aspect of the curve.

Avoiding zipping of the apex, ledge formation and transportation of the canal is difficult even for skilled hands; but, with practice and careful instrumentation, the effects can be minimized. Pre-curving instruments is an essential first line of defence. Upon insertion to their full length, instruments should be used in a filing action, and then very carefully. In this way, unfavourable pressures on the instruments can be avoided. The rotary action which is often used should be avoided at all costs, since this, more than any other act, is likely to generate a problem. Remember also that the stiffer the instrument (>No. 35) the more likely are the problems to occur. In this respect there is a particular problem in use of endosonic or other mechanized techniques, which tend to employ files that are generally stiffer than conventional hand instruments. They are mostly designed for use in the straight part of the canal, with hand instrumentation being used to complete the apical third and produce the apical stop. If their use is restricted to the straight part of the canal any untoward effects will be minimized.

Perforation or laceration

The most common form of perforation is seen apically, and is caused by filing beyond the working length. Perforation or laceration may also be due to difficulty in finding the canal during preparation of the access. They occasionally occur during preparation of the obturated canal for a post. Then it is the root-filling material, or perhaps a broken instrument within the canal, that is responsible for a deviation of the cutting instruments used in canal preparation. Perforation is far more likely to occur when engine-driven rotary instruments are used rather than hand instruments.

Perforation due to instrumentation where no post is required

Perforation at the time of canal preparation may take the form of apical trauma, with the possibility of extrusion of sealant into the apical tissues due to the lack of confinement during obturation. Tell-tale signs may include pain, discomfort and bleeding. Of course, prevention is better than cure; but if an apical perforation is suspected, first check, and if necessary re-establish a correct working length. Having done this, proceed to establish a new apical stop to the correct length. This will be straightforward if the original perforating instrument was of a small size. In the event that it was a large instrument it may be more difficult. In such cases dressing the canal for a week or two with calcium hydroxide paste may be indicated prior to the final obturation of the canal. In exceptional cases, an alternative, surgical approach may be needed.

Sometimes, in a multi-rooted tooth, perforation into the furcation occurs. This may be due to difficulty in finding root canals, or, occasionally, the result of over-preparation of already thin roots. The treatment of perforation in such cases is relatively straightforward, assuming that the perforation is not so severe as to require extraction of the tooth. The first action is to fill the canal with calcium hydroxide paste in the manner described earlier. After a suitable healing interval the canal can be obturated conventionally. Where the perforation is in the floor of the pulp chamber it may be sealed with glass–ionomer cement, after first inducing some healing by the application of calcium hydroxide paste. However, even after a successful repair the prognosis of the tooth must be guarded, and the patient should be advised accordingly.

Perforation due to post preparation

Commonly perforation occurs at the time of preparation of the canal for the post. This problem can be minimized if post preparation is carried out at the same visit as the obturation. Then the canal angulation and morphology is 'fresh' in the mind, and hence accidents are less likely. Further, if post preparation is left until the sealer has set, there is a risk of the seal being broken by the act of preparation. In all cases where the preparation is performed at a later visit or on a tooth obturated by another dentist, great care should be exercised.

In the event of perforation, there will usually be the tell-tale sign of bleeding and sensitivity or discomfort, assuming no local analgesia has been used. If this occurs, the post should never be definitively cemented. It is far better to seal the canal temporarily with a calcium hydroxide dressing. At a later visit, the canal can be re-entered and, after taking a check radiograph, an attempt can be made to realign the post. If this is possible, the post can be definitively cemented and the perforation dealt with via a surgical approach – assuming the location of the perforation is favourable. (A favourable perforation would be one which is accessible to the placement of a restoration after a flap has been reflected.) Unfavourable perforations are impossible to restore successfully after flap reflection, and are often located interproximally or palatally.

When the perforation is noted as an incidental finding on routine radiography, a decision has to be made about further treatment. Serial radiographs may be necessary to assess whether the associated lesion is static or changing. In the event that it is showing signs of enlargement it must be treated. A decision should first be made whether the post can be removed. If it is, a new post should be made in correct alignment with the canal, and the perforation should be dealt with via a surgical approach, using a standard buccal flap and carefully removing bone over the root until the perforation is located. In the event that it is impossible to remove the post, a surgical approach should be the primary option; but it is then often more difficult to effect a satisfactory repair to the perforation. Teeth which have been perforated have a diminished prognosis, and patients should be made aware of this. Nevertheless, with a careful technique and due attention paid to detail the prognosis for a favourable perforation is often excellent.

Summary

This chapter has considered some of the common problems which may be encountered with the endodontically treated tooth and some of the solutions to those problems. Whilst it cannot be all-embracing in such a limited space, it is hoped that the information contained is both practical and informative. For more detailed consideration, the reader is advised to consult the appropriate standard texts.

5

Periodontics

Keith Figures

Acute infections

Acute periodontal infections are not unusual in dental practice, but they are less common than infections arising from caries. As with any acute infection, painful symptoms develop rapidly and interfere with normal function. The symptoms may vary in severity, but treatment will usually be required and the patient will expect relief from pain. The conditions which can be considered as acute periodontal infections are:

- periodontal abscess
- acute necrotizing ulcerative gingivitis
- acute or primary herpetic gingivo-stomatitis
- pericoronitis
- infections with acute secondary periodontal symptoms.

Periodontal abscess

Periodontal abscesses are most frequently caused by the deep seeding of bacteria within the tissues, and it is important to remember that they may indicate a lowering of the host response. They can be acute or chronic, and the majority of periodontal abscesses, particularly if they have been inadequately treated, will be chronic for most of the time, with occasional acute flare-ups.

A periodontal abscess may be located in the soft tissues (for example, a gingival abscess due to an impacted toothbrush bristle) or in the deeper structures of the periodontal ligament. However, most commonly a periodontal abscess is found as an acute exacerbation of inflammation in a pre-existing periodontal pocket. (Nevertheless, periodontal abscesses do occur in apparently healthy areas following forceful penetration of foreign material into the tissue.) Precipitation of acute inflammation in existing pockets can be caused by food impaction due to, for example, lack of a contact point on a restoration, or retained gingival retraction cord after crown/bridge impressions; but probably the most common reason is where a scaling instrument punctures the pocket epithelium during scaling. For this reason the patient who has undergone root planing should always be warned of the possibility of a periodontal abscess developing in the days following treatment, and it may even be appropriate to consider antibiotics in some patients to prevent this happening.

All acute abscesses have certain symptoms in common. They usually develop rapidly, with the period from being first aware to the full-blown abscess often taking only a day. The pain from a typical abscess is felt as being 'deep and throbbing', with the severity depending on the tissue affected and its location. Generally, a gingival abscess is less painful than one affecting deeper structures. When the abscess involves the deeper aspects of the periodontal ligament it makes the tooth tender to biting or percussion, and often increases its mobility.

It is important to decide if the abscess is of periodontal or pulpal origin. A pulpal abscess is usually more painful, often keeping the patient awake at night. Thermal sensitivity may indicate the development of pulpitis; and, depending on the stage of pulpal degeneration, heat or cold application may relieve the pain or increase it. If the pulp is non-vital and there is a developing periapical abscess there will be no response to thermal change; this distinguishes it from a periodontal abscess where the pulp is vital. Secondly, the pain associated with a periodontal abscess is often easier for the patient to localize than pulpal pain. Pulpal pain can be diffuse and referred to the opposing arch; but as the inflammation reaches the periodontal ligament the pain starts to localize. Often a periapical radiograph clarifies the clinical picture, particularly if a GP point has been inserted into an associated sinus. The diagnosis can however be more difficult if a periodontal–endodontic lesion is present, and this case is covered later in this chapter.

In the acute phase the first step is to release pus, if it is present. As soon as the fluid pressure of the abscess is reduced the acute symptoms rapidly diminish. This can be achieved through the pocket's entrance in many cases, by inserting a periodontal probe, but will usually require local anaesthesia. If a fluctuant soft tissue swelling is evident this should be incised and drained under topical anaesthesia, such as ethyl chloride or xylocaine spray. Antimicrobials such as metronidazole or tetracycline may be prescribed over 5 days to ensure complete resolution of the infection. The patient can then return for pocket debridement, involving root planing and pocket irrigation with chlorhexidine. The ultrasonic scaler can be very useful here. The value of antimicrobial gels containing metronidazole (Elyzol) or minocycline (Dentomycin) that can be syringed into the pocket has yet to be established.

Acute necrotizing ulcerative gingivitis (ANUG)

This condition is not commonly seen these days, a fact that probably reflects improved levels of oral hygiene, decreased numbers of smokers and a generally more healthy diet. When it does occur it usually affects young adults, particularly those suffering from stress.

The clinical picture is characterized by extremely painful yellowish-white ulcers which begin on a few interdental papillae, bleed easily and destroy the papillary architecture. Halitosis is usual, and patients may complain of a metallic taste or that their teeth feel wedged apart. There is often a feeling of malaise, which is frequently accompanied by regional lymph node swelling. Once the acute phase has settled, particularly if treatment was not sought, the resulting poor gingival shape predisposes to further attacks, which encourage additional destruction of the gingival architecture. Patients with ANUG often have poor oral hygiene, which is frequently accompanied by a degree of personal neglect.

Analysis of patterns of distribution of ANUG has led most investigators to conclude that it is a non-communicable infectious disease of endogenous origin that cannot be transmitted from one person to another. There is no doubt that the clinical manifestations are caused by bacteria, since the condition rapidly responds to antibiotics. However, ANUG still remains a condition in which the specific organisms or combinations that produce the clinical manifestations have not been fully categorized.

The organisms that have been isolated from the ulcers of ANUG are *Treponema vincenti* and *Fusobacterium fusiformis*, together with various black-pigmenting organisms, including *Prevotella intermedia* (*Bacteroides intermedius*) and *Prevotella intermelaninogenica* (*Bacteroides melaninogenicus*). The significance of these organisms in the disease process is as yet unknown. It is agreed that, although ANUG is an anaerobic infection by organisms which invade the host tissue, it usually responds to local treatment. Renewed interest in ANUG has arisen recently because of its occurrence in people who are HIV-positive. It is important to bear in mind that this condition may be responsible for the development of ANUG in an apparently healthy young individual. It is seen in the HIV-positive individual as one of the later manifestations of HIV infection. In common with some of the other oral complications that may be seen in this condition, HIV-associated ANUG represents a further

Table 5.1 Staging of HIV infection based on the Walter Reed classification

Stage	*Criteria*
Stage 0	Contact with HIV
Stage 1	Transient episodes of fever, antibodies to HIV detected
Stage 2	Persistent lymphadenopathy often present for many months
Stage 3	Drop in level of circulating T4 cells to about 50% of normal
Stage 4	T4 cells depleted, other immune defects become apparent
Stage 5	T4 cells depleted, oral infections and complications develop
Stage 6	Generalized opportunistic infections evident, onset of full-blown AIDS

deterioration in the patient's health, and indicates that at some stage in the near future full-blown AIDS will develop.

A classification of HIV infection developed from the original designed by the Walter Reed Army Institute of Dental Research, Washington, DC (Redfield *et al.* 1986) is shown in **Table 5.1** and reproduced with permission from the *New England Journal of Medicine.*

Six stages are distinguished in **Table 5.1:**

1 There are no clear symptoms at this stage, but HIV antibodies are present.
2 Chronic lymph node swelling is evident, often of several months duration.
3 There are immune system disturbances and a drop in the number of circulating T4 lymphocytes. The duration of this stage can be up to 2 years.
4 A skin test for delayed hypersensitivity reveals a poor reaction. This phase may last for 2 years.
5 The dentist may see HIV-associated periodontal disease and evidence of fungal, bacterial or viral infections. The most likely bacterial infection is ANUG-associated gingivitis/periodontitis. In addition, hairy leukoplakia may be apparent, and similarly, Kaposi's sarcoma. A skin test for delayed hypersensitivity is negative. This phase may 'ast for 1–2 years.
6 Severe immune deficiency is present (AIDS), together with opportunistic infections, severe periodontal disease and tumour formation. Most patients die within 2 years.

Many therapeutic agents have been found to relieve the symptoms of ANUG successfully. Nevertheless, in most cases local debridement using an ultrasonic scaler combined with improved home mouth care is effective; but if systemic upset is evident a course of metronidazole, 200 mg three times a day for three days, is indicated. The use of a sodium perborate mouthwash (e.g. Bocasan) can often be useful in the acute phase. If an ultrasonic scaling is necessary then to reduce aerosol bacterial loading it is advisable to ask the patient to first rinse with a 0.2 per cent chlorhexidine gluconate mouthwash before starting. Chlorhexidine can also be recommended for home use to improve oral hygiene more quickly. In the longer term, and when oral hygiene permits, gingivoplasty may be required to improve gingival contour.

Acute or primary herpetic gingivostomatitis

This condition can usually be diagnosed without difficulty, as the history, signs and symptoms are characteristic. Typically the patient is a child 1–6 years old or a young adult who has been unwell and pyrexic for 2–4 days, who then develops an extremely sore mouth, with ulcers ranging from 1–4 mm in diameter on the gingivae and oral mucosa generally. In addition to the fever, which may rise to 40° C, there is often pallor, nausea, lymph node involvement and pharyngitis. Not surprisingly, there is also a loss of appetite, and all oral hygiene practices will have ceased. The disease usually runs its course in 10–14 days, with the systemic symptoms starting to disappear in 7–10 days. Unless the patient is immunocompromised healing will be complete in 14 days, leaving no evidence of prior infection.

The cause is *Herpes simplex* virus. Epidemiological studies show that 80 per cent of the population harbour the virus in the deep epithelial tissues and have specific antibodies against it. There are two distinct strains of this DNA virus: Type 1 causes acute herpetic gingivostomatitis and recurrent herpes labialis, while Type 2 is usually found in, and recovered from, the genital areas, and is transmitted by sexual contact. It is possible for the Type 2 infection to present orally as a primary manifestation. The primary manifestation of the Type 1 infection is usually seen in children, but can be seen in people who are in their twenties. It is contagious, and the incubation period before the clinical symptoms become apparent is 7 days. Only about 5 per cent of patients are systemically affected, and hence are quite ill. The other 95 per cent contract the disease asymptomatically, and show no signs of illness.

Treatment

When children are suffering from this condition it is important to reassure parents and advise carefully on treatment. Topical analgesia such as Xylocaine Ointment 5 per cent will help to reduce the discomfort of the ulcers, particularly at meal times (if it can be applied!). In addition, a soft diet can be recommended, along with increased fluid intake. Such a diet may include cold milk and water, together with cool yoghurts, custard and ice cream. Analgesics such as paracetamol elixir or ibuprofen (for patients over 12 years) control the pyrexia, and plenty of rest on a warm couch in front of the TV is advisable. Reassurance and an explanation that the disease will need to run its course should be given to all patients with symptoms. Chlorhexidine mouthwash helps to keep plaque levels down and reduce the secondary infection of the ulcers, and in children it may help to swab the mouth with chlorhexidine on a cotton bud or a small mouth sponge. Severely ill or immunocompromised patients should receive systemic Acyclovir, and should be under the care of a physician.

It is as well to warn the parents of the highly contagious nature of this condition, and that other young family members and friends may become infected. It is also possible for vesicles to form on the fingers or thumbs, particularly if the child is in the habit of digit-sucking.

Pericoronitis

This is particularly common in young adults with erupting third molars, but can occur during the eruption of other teeth. The most commonly recommended treatment is irrigation underneath the operculum with 0.2 per cent chlorhexidine gluconate and prescription of a five-day course of an antibiotic such as metronidazole, which is effective against the anaerobic organisms often implicated in pericoronitis. The removal of the opposing third molar also allows the inflamed operculum to resolve more rapidly by eliminating any occlusal trauma. Ultimately, removal of the erupting/impacted third molar is indicated, particularly if there is no attached gingiva distal to this tooth.

Occasionally, patients present with pericoronitis as an oral manifestation of an underlying systemic condition. When pericoronitis is bilateral it may indicate that the immune response is somewhat depressed, and it may be worthwhile to perform haematological investigations, such as a full blood count (FBC) together with Haemoglobin (Hb). This might be undertaken more easily in conjunction with the local medical practitioner; and a telephone call to the medical practice to discuss the case and the most appropriate tests is advisable. Futhermore, young adults are susceptible to infectious mononucleosis, which could also be the reason for the pericoronitis being persistent and/or bilateral; here again liaison with the medical practitioner is advisable.

Surgical removal of the operculum is indicated after the acute phase has settled in some cases. The sort of case where an operculectomy may be tried is where the tooth is nearly erupted (into a good occlusion) and there is sufficient space in the retromolar region to accommodate the crown. This can be performed most easily using an electrosurgery unit, thus often avoiding the need for suturing. However, this type of surgical procedure is not always successful, and ultimately the tooth may need removing.

Acute systemic conditions with secondary periodontal symptoms

Chicken pox (varicella virus) can produce small vesicles on the gingivae which burst to become ulcers. It is caused by the same virus which causes herpes zoster, and the oral lesions are very similar in both conditions. The prevalence of tuberculosis is increasing again, and there are reports in the literature of tuberculous gingivitis. Tuberculous ulcers in the mouth are very painful, and slowly increase in size with the passage of time. They may be found in areas of trauma, and should not be confused with traumatic ulcers. Tuberculosis is more common in people from ethnic minorities, who may have developed it abroad, and also in those who are homeless; in such patients it should always be considered in the differential diagnosis of painful oral ulceration. Furthermore, patients who carry the HIV virus are more susceptible to tuberculosis.

Two cases seen by the author which demonstrate a need for vigilance regarding an underlying systemic condition are described below.

Case 1

The patient was a 34-year-old postman referred by his general dental practitioner, who had performed a scaling on the previous day. The patient still suffered from persistent mild bleeding from between the upper central incisors. Examination revealed an apparently healthy individual without signs of systemic illness, but who had slight bleeding between the upper central incisors. This was arrested by applying a periodontal dressing (Coepak), and the patient was sent for blood tests to screen for an underlying problem. The report was quickly returned from the haematologist as being an atypical form of acute leukaemia, and treatment was started immediately. Unfortunately, the patient's condition did not respond to therapy, and he died 3 weeks later.

Case 2

The patient was a 54-year-old woman who presented as a dental emergency complaining of bleeding from the gingiva between the 36 and 37. This had been present for 24 hours, and she had been unable to stop it. It had occurred spontaneously, and was not profuse, but a persistent ooze. Examination revealed the patient to be overweight and to have a ruddy complexion. Intraorally she had moderate oral hygiene, and an overhang was present on a restoration in 36. The bleeding was again arrested using a Coepak dressing. Further questioning of the patient's male companion revealed that she consumed a half-bottle of sherry each day! As a result of this information she was referred to a consultant physician, where liver function tests revealed her liver metabolism to be abnormal, and hence affecting clotting function. Corrective therapy for alcohol abuse was started, and in due course her own GDP corrected her dental condition.

Dentine sensitivity

Dentine sensitivity is the term used for pain arising from exposed dentine, typically in response to thermal, chemical or osmotic stimuli, and is often associated with gingival recession or root abrasion, which of course may occur after successful periodontal therapy. The prevalence of dentine sensitivity is likely to increase because:

- More adults will be keeping their teeth in the future.
- Gingival recession will become more prevalent, as will the number of exposed root surfaces.
- As people become more dentally aware the incidence of tooth wear due to destructive brushing techniques will increase.

The aetiology of dentine sensitivity is still obscure, although various theories have been proposed. That most commonly accepted is the hydrodynamic theory, which suggests that fluid movement within the dentinal tubules is the likely source of disturbance within dentine. This disturbance or displacement of fluid is detected by nerve endings in peripulpal dentine and interpreted as pain. Research has shown that if many open dentinal tubules are present on the exposed dentine surface, and if these tubules have a large tubule diameter, then the chance of significant fluid flow within each tubule is greater.

It appears that changes at the dentine surface are important in determining dentine sensitivity. This is based on the fact that patients experiencing sensitivity can be divided into two categories: those experiencing sharp unexpected pain in an isolated site, and those who suffer a more generalized level of pain varying in intensity as time passes. In this second group it is possible to see a balance developing between factors tending to occlude dentine tubules (use of desensitizing toothpastes and topically applied agents, such as a fluoride varnish like Duraphat) and factors tending to open them, like acidic foods, citrus fruits, fizzy drinks, etc.

Structural changes seen in dentine after acid exposure

When dentine is cut or abraded a smear layer forms on the surface, which occludes the tubules and can only be removed by acid etching. Research has shown that the smear layer can be removed by acids present in some foods and also in acidic drinks. In addition, the openings of the tubules at the etched or cut dentine surface are enlarged, and this renders the dentine more susceptible to external influences. Therefore dietary factors may play an important part in increasing the sensitivity of exposed dentine by opening up large numbers of tubules.

Approaches to treatment

There are two ways to reduce the discomfort of exposed sensitive dentine: namely, either to interfere with sensory nerve function directly, or alternatively to occlude the tubules. In studies where deep cavities were cut in dentine, solutions rich in potassium ions have been shown to be very effective in inhibiting sensory nerve activity. This may help explain the success of desensitizing toothpastes containing potassium salts (for example, Sensodyne F).

However, a more predictable and quicker means of reducing dentine sensitivity is to occlude the tubules. Patients with this condition often try to reduce their symptoms by using one of the desensitizing toothpastes. These dentifrices have a variety of ingredients which, it is claimed, will induce tubule occlusion. Recent research has shown one of these ingredients in particular to be very effective in occluding tubules. The effective ingredient was silica; and it subsequently transpired that its effectiveness could be enhanced by strontium ions. Additional research has shown that when tubules are occluded by silica the presence of water (or saliva) does not disrupt the blockage formed at the end of the tubule.

Prevention of sensitivity

The pain from exposed root dentine does not occur as an isolated event, but as discomfort, which increases in intensity with the passage of time. Clinical techniques which aim to stop this

Table 5.2 Differential diagnosis of dentine sensitivity

Cracked tooth syndrome
Chipped tooth
Fractured restoration
Caries (primary or secondary)
Progressive pulpitis (e.g. under a crown)
Occlusal trauma

progressive increase in discomfort include dietary analysis and modification, and correction of any faults in toothbrushing technique.

There is strong evidence that diet can have a marked effect on the incidence of pain from exposed dentine. This is particularly true if the diet contains acid components. If this intake can be curtailed then the surface of the dentine should be more conducive to the formation of a surface smear layer and, as already shown, this should reduce the chances of fluid movement within each dentinal tubule.

The importance of a toothbrushing technique to minimize destruction appears obvious. A destructive technique which induces gingival recession must be corrected; but this should be balanced with the need to establish a dentine smear layer using the silica components of the toothpaste. Therefore it is recommended that patients brush before rather than after meals, particularly if a dietary acid will be present (for example, fruit juice with breakfast, wine with a meal). Brushing after a meal containing acid elements is more likely to accelerate the erosion of enamel and dentine, and possibly to open more tubules in areas of exposed root dentine.

By brushing before a meal the pH in the mouth will be kept neutral and plaque activity will be reduced, and the chances of creating an insulating smear layer on the dentine are probably increased.

Management of sensitivity

Dentine sensitivity can be frustrating to treat. As with any new patient, a full history is required before a diagnosis is made. A patient with a neglected mouth may have several possible sources of pain, and it should be explained that treatment may not provide an instant solution to the discomfort. For comparison other causes of pulpal stimulation that simulate dentine sensitivity are shown in **Table 5.2**.

When the diagnosis is confirmed there are two ways to treat the condition. One involves using any of the available techniques to seal the dentinal tubules. A few applications of one of the following materials might help:

- fluoride-containing varnish
- glass–ionomer cement
- dentine adhesives
- resin.

The other technique is brushing with a desensitizing dentifrice. This will not produce a rapid reduction in pain levels, and in some patients will not satisfy their demand for pain relief. It should be pointed out that it will take some time to achieve relief – sometimes 3–4 weeks. For this approach to achieve success advice must be given on diet at the same time as information on brushing. If after 3–4 weeks' use the levels of sensitivity are decreasing then brushing with a regular dentifrice may be resumed. Patients should be warned, however, that if discomfort on brushing returns, further use of the desensitizing dentifrice is needed. If the discomfort does not resolve as a result of this approach the dentist should suspect another cause (cracked tooth, caries). If no other cause can be found a tubule-sealing technique should be applied to the sensitive area(s).

Fluoride treatment

For patients whose sensitivity persists following initial use of a desensitizing toothpaste an alternative fluoride treatment can be considered. For a long time fluoride has been found to be useful in such circumstances. The exact mechanism of action is uncertain, but it is thought to increase the stability of the dentine surface by making it less soluble in acid. Also in concentrations of around 2 per cent it has been shown that calcium fluoride forms, which occludes the tubule. The possible fluoride treatments that may be appropriate for sensitivity include:

- a daily rinse with 0.05 per cent sodium fluoride mouth rinse
- regular use of a fluoride dentifrice
- application of an alcoholic varnish containing 2.26 per cent fluoride (Duraphat)
- application of a synthetic varnish containing 12 per cent fluoride (Bifluorid 12, Voco, Cuxhaven, Germany)

Final solution treatments

If the sensitivity persists after trying the above alternatives and there is no other detectable cause for the pain then the penultimate solution is to prepare a shallow cavity and restore with glass–ionomer cement. This should prevent any further trouble; but occasionally even this does not help, and then the only alternative is to extirpate the pulp or extract the tooth.

Traumatic and chemical damage

Trauma to the oral tissues can be due to a number of causes. Acute injury due to the impact of a solid structure (like a fist) will in all probability damage teeth and alveolar bone as well as gingiva, and all these structures will need treatment. However, it is possible for some types of injury to peel gingiva away from bone, rather like what happens in reflecting a dental flap. This is usually due to a hard structure (like a steering wheel) hitting the teeth at an angle and then sliding apically, taking the gingiva with it. These injuries can often be quite easily repaired by careful suturing, after a good debridement to remove any foreign material. An anti-tetanus injection and a course of appropriate antibiotics should be given to all patients with injuries of this type.

Gingival tissue damage is much more likely to occur as a result of poor clinical dentistry. Examples include poor marginal adaptation of crowns which are extended subgingivally: overhanging margins on approximal restorations will initially cause localized inflammation and eventually lead to pocket formation. Careless use of dental burs can abrade gingival tissues, and when this occurs it is advisable to recommend an antiseptic mouthwash like chlorhexidine for a few days post-operatively to minimize plaque collection in the area. Poorly designed tissue-borne partial dentures can cause stripping of gingival tissue on abutment teeth, particularly if the acrylic flash has not been eased from the gingival fitting area of the denture. The incomplete removal of gingival retraction cord after impression-taking can be another reason for persistent gingival inflammation. This in turn can lead to gingival abscess formation, which sometimes develops a few days after impressions were taken. Tears of the gingiva after an extraction are always sutured to ensure good gingival healing.

One unusual example of gingival trauma is gingivitis artifacta. In this condition the patient presents with a traumatic lesion for which there is no obvious dental cause. Self-inflicted trauma is not always easy to detect, but should be suspected if the patient has an unusual pattern of gingival stripping that cannot be explained by poor toothbrushing technique. These patients are often of a highly nervous disposition, and produce the gingival condition by picking at the gingival margins with their finger nails or some other implement. Referral to the medical practitioner for counselling may be the course to follow if this is suspected. Another type of injury may be seen in the patient who induces gingival damage by the over-zealous use of dental floss. Typically this causes abrasion or cutting of the interdental papilla, and may be seen either in an isolated area or more generally in the mouth.

Chemical trauma

One of the commonest causes of chemical trauma to the gingival tissues is an aspirin burn as a result of the patient's placing an aspirin tablet next to a painful tooth. This produces necrotic sloughing of the gingival tissues in the area of contact, with lifting of the superficial layers of epithelium, producing a white appearance of the mucosa. This can be produced after holding the tablet in the area for only an hour or so.

Nevertheless, other forms of chemical trauma do still occur, and are usually due to poorly performed dental procedures. Causes include acid etchant burning the gingiva or hydrogen peroxide used for bleaching a tooth that has spread on to the gingiva. The increasing use of rubber dams in dentistry will help to prevent these accidents.

Another more unusual cause of chemical trauma is hypersensitivity to a dental material. An example is the patient who is allergic to methyl methacrylate monomer, and has recently had a temporary acrylic crown cemented. This produces a quite marked gingival inflammation locally, and can be quite uncomfortable for the patient, particularly if gingival trauma occurred during the crown preparation, allowing the irritant effect to be more pronounced. It is also possible for some luting cements to producc inflammation; but the most likely cause here is plaque collection on the overhanging cement margins, which may not have been trimmed away correctly.

The periodontic–endodontic lesion

Acute inflammatory changes in the vital pulp rarely produce clinically detectable changes in the periodontal tissues. A tooth with pulpitis may occasionally be associated with radiographic signs of inflammation such as widening of the apical periodontal ligament space; whereas a tooth with a non-vital pulp frequently shows involvement of the periodontal ligament space. In the necrotic pulp micro-organisms find conditions which encourage their growth. These bacteria may grow on necrotic material or exudates which have formed in the root canal or on the canal walls, where they often penetrate the dentinal tubules.

The bacteria found in necrotic pulps share many features with the bacteria found in periodontal disease. The vast majority of these bacteria are anaerobes; but there are also spirochetes and motile organisms present. As these bacteria proliferate they release exotoxins, which ultimately reach the periodontal ligament via various canals and foramina that connect the pulp chamber with the periodontal ligament. Once inflammatory changes are initiated, periodontal ligament fibres are destroyed, along with adjacent alveolar bone. This occurs most commonly around the apex of a tooth. The amount of tissue destruction seen is dependent on the number and virulence of the bacteria present, but also on the ability of the host to limit the spread of infection. When a balanced host–bacterial relationship is established the involved site may remain quiescent and unchanged in size for years. At the other end of the spectrum, cyst development may occur, and result in extensive long-term bone destruction.

Difficulties in diagnosing the causes of deep vertical bone loss localized to a single tooth, which is often a sign of a periodontic–endodontic lesion and commonly due to the presence of accessory canals, are evident. The clinician has to answer the question: is this lesion due to a necrotic pulp that has spread via an accessory canal to involve the gingival margin, or is it due to periodontitis that has progressed apically to involve the furcation? In addition, it should be recalled which paths of communication exist between the pulp and the periodontal ligament. Possibilities include:

- accessory canals – usually in the apical third of the root but often in the furcation of molar teeth
- dentinal tubules
- iatrogenic perforations (post and core, endodontics, pins).

Associated radiographic features

These include deep restorations, evidence of attempts at endodontic treatment, caries reaching the pulp, root perforation due to poor technique when preparing for a post crown, and an isolated vertical

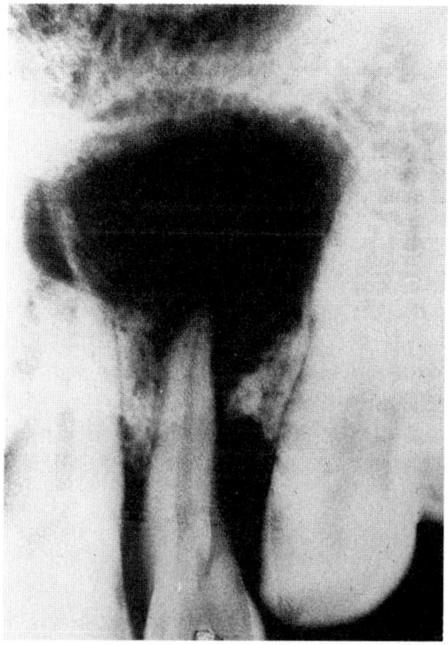

Figure 5.1 Periodontal disease resulting in marked bone loss has exposed a distal palatal groove, resulting in secondary pulpal involvement.

bone defect in the furcation or in the apical third of the root. The diagnosis of perio–endo lesions can be considered under three headings:

- primarily arising from a necrotic pulp with secondary periodontal involvement
- primarily arising from the periodontal tissues with secondary pulpal involvement (see Figure 5.1)
- true combined lesions where the original cause of the bone loss is obscure. (Here the root canal and pocket are in communication, and support a similar microbial population.)

Treatment

Endodontic therapy is the first line of treatment when the tooth is found to be non-vital. This may have to be prolonged as a result of repeated reinfection of the root canal from the pocket. Successful root filling of the tooth allows the bone defect to heal. The prognosis for multirooted teeth with furcation involvement depends on the following factors:

- the extent of horizontal and vertical bone loss in the furcation area
- the number of roots and their morphology
- the amount of remaining periodontal support
- the chances of successful endodontics
- the chances of successful surgical correction
- the mental and physical ability of the patient to cope with the often prolonged treatment and possibly complicated after-care

If the periodontal defect persists after effective sealing of the root canal, this must be treated by conventional periodontal techniques such as scaling and root planing. If this is still unsuccessful then root resection of a multirooted tooth may be indicated, or indeed tunnel preparation to produce a 'through and through' defect that the patient can clean with a bottle brush. If all else fails the final solution is to extract.

The management of post-surgical pain

The amount of periodontal surgery now performed is considerably less than it used to be. Generally, the level of postoperative discomfort is not great after periodontal surgery. Post-operative pain is most likely to occur after gingivectomy or where bone removal has taken place. The regular use of non-specific anti-inflammatory drugs will suffice in the majority of cases, and patients should be advised to use the analgesic they commonly have available at home. Pain normally settles after a few days; but if it increases in intensity this may indicate that an infection is developing, particularly if systemic signs are present. Antibiotics will then be required, and the use of metronidazole 400 mg twice daily for 5 days is recommended, as the vast majority of infections will be anaerobic in nature. (When prescribing metronidazole, or indeed other antibiotics to women taking the oral contraceptive pill, they should be advised that the efficiency of 'the pill' may be impaired, and that the use of additional contraceptive methods is appropriate.) If a periodontal dressing has been placed it should be removed to allow proper inspection of the surgical site and allow for the drainage of any pus present. The use of chlorhexidine mouthwash in all patients who have had surgery is recommended, to keep plaque retention to a minimum during the healing period.

Concluding remarks

There are of course other conditions that can affect the periodontal tissues, such as lichen planus or the bullous conditions that occasionally present in the mouth. They are not very common in practice, and are not covered here, particularly as treatment in most cases would require specialist help. Nevertheless, when such patients are in remission supervision by a member of the dental practice team may be appropriate, and treatment in all probability would be aimed at keeping plaque levels low, using a careful brushing technique. The hospital consultant would be happy to involve the practitioner in the care of these cases where possible, and a telephone call indicating this could be beneficial to all concerned.

6

Paediatric dentistry

Lesley E. Davidson

Introduction

Since the introduction of capitation there has been a steady increase in the number of children registered for treatment or advice with general dental practitioners. Even so, children frequently arrive with injuries or acute infections, and the increasing proportion of children receiving active orthodontic care can experience problems with fixed or removable appliances. Therefore, despite a steady improvement in the oral health of children, emergencies can arise and distressed children often arrive unannounced, at an inconvenient time, accompanied by an anxious adult. Remember that at these times it is the dental need of the child which is paramount.

Acute infection from dental causes

Deciduous dentition

Infection of the pulp is most frequently caused by caries. A less frequent occurrence is exposure of the pulp following trauma or as a result of restorative procedures. Tooth wear, most commonly due to erosion, is increasingly a cause of pulpal complications.

The morphology of a primary molar tooth renders the pulp considerably more vulnerable to bacterial attack than that of its permanent successor, and both coronal and radicular portions can be rapidly destroyed. The resulting inflammation may remain sub-acute or chronic, giving the patient little or no pain, but having the potential to flare into an acute infection at any time.

Abscesses are much more common in primary molars than in primary anterior teeth. The crown morphology renders them more susceptible to carious attack, initially in the fissures or just below the large interproximal contact areas. Furthermore, they remain in the mouth for a decade, while deciduous anterior teeth are normally shed after a much shorter period.

Diagnosis

Provided that the history reveals no systemic complications which take precedence and govern the treatment which can be provided, when a young child presents with pain or swelling two decisions have to be made: which tooth is causing the problem and whether there is pulpal involvement. Identifying the cause of the problem may be difficult if there are several carious, worn, traumatized or heavily restored teeth. Since the pulpal histology is not readily apparent, the clinician has to rely on other evidence, by pooling information from the history, clinical examination and radiographs.

Presentation with intermittent pain is unusual in the deciduous dentition. The effect of hot and cold or sweet substances may indicate an underlying pulpal hyperaemia. Excavation of the carious lesion followed by a sedative dressing such as zinc oxide/eugenol should suffice. This procedure however should not be undertaken to avoid management problems or in the mistaken belief that it will work when there is a history of spontaneous or continued pain.

Spontaneous pain, especially if sufficiently severe to keep the child awake at night or to require analgesics, is likely to indicate advanced pulpal involvement, and it is then necessary to decide whether or not the tooth is vital. If on examination there is intra- or extra-oral swelling or a sinus, the pulp is probably dead. There may only be redness or soreness of the mucosa, usually on the buccal side of the suspect tooth. Further investigation by percussion of teeth is not a patient-friendly test in children, and is best avoided. Nevertheless, increased mobility of a tooth over and above that which would be expected for the patient's age, or as compared with its antimere, is a particularly useful sign of infection.

Caries usually starts interproximally once the contact points close, and therefore bitewings should be taken routinely. These may well reveal intra-radicular radiolucencies or internal resorption, either of which would confirm the diagnosis and in addition provide valuable information regarding the rest of the dentition. To improve co-operation when taking bitewings, small periapical radiographs, for example, Kodak size O ($^7/_8$″ × $1^3/_4$″) are best, and are well tolerated in small mouths, especially when the corners are eased. The use of E speed film reduces the time and exposure necessary.

Treatment

At presentation the immediate priority is for pain relief. Often the child will be accompanied by an adult, who narrates a history of pain at night resulting in both the child and the parents losing sleep.

The adult may well expect marvels to be performed, and this in turn tends to put pressure on the practitioner. However, quite commonly after one or two disturbed nights the child may no longer be in pain; and it is then important to bear in mind who is being treated.

The appearance of an associated swelling is dramatic; but commonly the pain will have subsided with its onset. Assuming the medical history does not limit the clinical options, the immediate treatment is to effect drainage. Either extract the offending tooth or, using hand instruments, open up the tooth and remove the necrotic pulp.

If the child has a pronounced swelling and is pyrexic, systemic antibiotics can be prescribed – usually Amoxycillin (child up to 10 years – 125 mg 3 times a day for 5 days; over 10 years – 250 mg 3 times a day for 5 days, after a double loading dose. Metronidazole (3 to 7 years) by weight but 100 mg twice daily for 5 days; 7 to 10 years 100 g 3 times a day for 5 days may be used in conjunction with this, with the usual exceptions for those who are allergic. If an elixir is given, this should be in sugar-free form. For pain relief, paracetamol, either in tablet or as sugar-free elixir (1–5 years, 120–250 mg; 6–12 years, 250–500 mg, maximum 4 times a day) may be recommended.

Clearly if there is pyrexia and pronounced swelling that might lead to a spreading infection, extractions under general anaesthesia may be considered. If the airway is thought to be at risk the patient should be admitted to hospital. However, local drainage should be the first recourse, and will usually suffice for the immediate situation, so allowing the operator time to consider the long-term management.

If a sinus is present which allows drainage, then, providing that co-operation allows, the tooth can be dressed with an appropriate disinfectant after removal of the necrotic pulp remnants. Beechwood creosote is still the most successful medicament. This is applied on a small pledget of cotton wool inserted without pressure into the cavity and sealed with a zinc oxide/eugenol temporary dressing. A subsequent appointment in approximately 10 days' time should be made for completion of the restoration.

Where there is spontaneous pain but no swelling or sinus, the condition of the pulp and its vitality is less certain. In these situations, local analgesia is essential, and should be given at the outset. To aid this, surface anaesthetics are routinely used, and are available in a variety of flavours, such as pina-colada, bubble-gum, creme-de-menthe, cinnamon and rum butter, as well as the more traditional mint. Lower deciduous anteriors and all teeth in the upper arch can be anaesthetized by infiltration. Half a cartridge of local anaesthetic solution (lignocaine 2 per cent with 1/80 000 adrenaline) is delivered by the smallest gauge needle suitable. A 19 mm 30 gauge short needle has sufficient length for infiltration and is narrower than the 36 mm 27 gauge needle necessary for an inferior dental block. In the lower arch, a buccal infiltration for the lower second deciduous molar is effective up to about 4 or 5 years of age, and for the lower first deciduous molar until 5 or 6 years of age. For the older child, this may be supplemented by intraligamentary anaesthesia; or alternatively an inferior alveolar nerve block will achieve the profound anaesthesia necessary.

In deciduous incisors with their straight, short, wide canals pulpectomy is the treatment of choice, and canal obturation is with a resorbable material like calcium hydroxide or iodoform paste (iodoform 80 per cent, parachlorophenol 2.025 per cent, camphor 4.8 per cent and menthol 1.21 per cent). For deciduous molars, however, pulpotomy will be necessary, since their canal morphology precludes more conventional root canal treatment. The exposure of an empty pulp chamber or one containing granular debris indicates dry necrosis, whilst the presence of pus clearly indicates that the tooth is non-vital. In either case beechwood creosote is applied.

When there is profuse haemorrhage from the radicular pulp, treatment should proceed by application of a mummifying dressing of formocresol. This may be carried on a portion of cotton wool pledget and applied to the remaining pulp stumps for 5 minutes. If this proves impossible, the dressing may be placed in the pulp chamber and sealed with a temporary dressing for a week. Formocresol is available in proprietary form or can be made up by a pharmacist to Buckley's original formula (formalin 19 ml, cresol 35 ml, glycerine 25 ml, water 21 ml). Care should be taken in its application, since it is extremely caustic. However, with this technique clinical success rates are good.

When extractions are needed, it is important to bear in mind the principal recommendation of a recent report on general anaesthesia (Poswillo Report, 1990) that 'the use of general anaesthesia should be avoided wherever possible'. It is crucial to avoid repeated general anaesthetics for the same patient. Bearing in mind the probably symmetrical nature of the carious process, the need to remove other teeth of poor prognosis as well as the need to balance deciduous canine and first molar extractions, should be taken into account.

Permanent dentition

In permanent teeth the most likely cause of pulpal infection in a molar is caries, while infection in anteriors is more likely to be due to trauma. Immediate treatment should be directed to pain relief, with subsequent visits for the definitive treatment taking into account the long-term overall plan for tooth, mouth and child.

Diagnosis

Acute infection is still most successfully diagnosed by consideration of the symptoms of sinus, swelling or tenderness, tooth discoloration and/or mobility, combined with radiographic evidence of apical radiolucency. In this context it is important to remember that the position of the 'apex' of an immature incisor may well be only a few millimetres subgingival, with the attendant swelling or sinus mimicking the presentation of a periodontal abscess.

Pulp vitality testing in children is frequently unreliable and can give ambiguous results, in part because children may be uncooperative, but also because immature teeth respond inconsistently. Following trauma, further confusion occurs, because a negative response may be a consequence of a damaged nerve supply rather than a defective blood supply.

Molar teeth

The first permanent molar is the tooth most commonly affected by caries, where it is sometimes superimposed on existing hypoplasia. In 1993, more than half of children 12 or more years old had carious first molar teeth. As a result it may sometimes be necessary to consider extraction of first permanent molar teeth. Classically the best age for this is between $8^1/_2$ and 10 years of age, when up to a third of children are affected. Full consideration must then be given to minimizing undesirable effects on the occlusion by appropriate balancing and/or compensating extractions. Should a younger child present with symptoms, it may prove necessary to restore the diseased tooth temporarily until an age more suitable for planned extraction.

Assuming that the tooth is to be saved, the primary aim must be to maintain vitality in order to ensure complete root development. Following administration of analgesia the tooth should be isolated, caries should be removed and the pulp should be protected by indirect or direct pulp capping with calcium hydroxide and sealed with zinc oxide/eugenol cement. At a subsequent appointment, a permanent restoration can be inserted, provided that symptoms have resolved.

Unfortunately, a painful, hyperaemic pulp is commonly found to result in a carious exposure. Assuming that adequate anaesthesia has been achieved and provided that the exposure is small (involving only a pulp horn) direct pulp capping with calcium hydroxide may suffice. Where symptoms persist and when it is essential to retain this particular tooth – for example, when the adjacent second premolar is absent and there is as yet no evidence of a third molar – conventional root canal treatment is the only solution. This is only possible when the tooth is fully developed with closed apices. In those situations where the first permanent molar exhibits incomplete root development pulpotomy is the intermediate treatment of choice, using calcium hydroxide as the base lining in order to promote root completion.

Anterior teeth

Anterior teeth, usually upper incisors, may become non-vital as a result of trauma, developmental anomaly, erosion or, less frequently of late, through caries. Pulpal damage usually occurs either through disruption of the blood supply or by frank exposure of the pulp. In addition, when exposed dentinal tubules remain patent, bacterial contamination may advance to the pulp. The Children's Dental Health Survey (O'Brien, 1995) noted that 70–96 per cent of traumatized anterior teeth had remained untreated, and those with problems other than enamel failure were therefore at risk.

The non-vital tooth should be isolated, preferably by the use of a rubber dam, and access gained either through the fracture line, if traumatized and unrestored, or through the palatal surface of the tooth. It should be remembered that in some instances the tooth may be only part-erupted and access may need to be further gingival than when encountered in mature dentitions. In view of the width of an immature tooth root canal, the pulp should be extirpated using two or three barbed broaches rotated around one another.

Having established a working length radiographically and after appropriate filing, the canal should be irrigated, dried and filled to the apex with a radiopaque non-setting calcium hydroxide paste. This is available in syringe form (e.g. 'Reogan Rapid', Vivadent, Lichtenstein; 'Pulpdent', Pulpdent Corp., Waterman, US). Alternatively, calcium hydroxide can be spun into the canal using a rotary paste filler; be introduced via a jiffy tube; or be persuaded into place with the blunt end of a paper point. Follow-up treatment depends on whether the tooth is immature, with an open apex, or is fully formed. In the former, treatment is aimed at allowing 'apexification' to continue and ultimately at being able to place a conventional root canal filling.

Very occasionally extraction may be considered, for instance in the case of malformed upper lateral incisors. Careful consideration should then be given to the status of the contralateral tooth if present. Naturally it is better to instigate emergency treatment for the tooth in the first instance, in order that long-term decisions, possibly after discussion with an orthodontist, can be effected in a controlled manner.

Acute systemic infections with oral manifestations

Systemic viral infections are common in infancy and childhood, and the dentist should be familiar with their manifestations.

Acute herpetic gingivostomatitis

This condition is described in Chapter 5.

Herpangina

This infection is caused by a Coxsackie virus, occurs in young children of approximately 6 to 7 years of age, and is far less severe than herpetic gingivostomatitis. The child is usually ill for 3 to 5 days. Vesicles similar to those of primary herpes appear, but are restricted more to the throat and soft palate. The gingivae remain unaffected. There is a mild pyrexia, and often a history of sore throat preceding the vesicles/ulceration.

Treatment

Again treatment is restricted to supportive therapy, and consists largely of reassuring the parents that the child is not seriously ill and that the disease will run its course. A soft or liquid diet containing adequate fluids is recommended, supplemented with analgesics. Healing occurs rapidly within 3 or 4 days. Arrangements should be made to review the child after a suitable interval to ensure that healing has occurred.

Hand, foot and mouth disease

Children with this viral infection (caused by Coxsackie A16) are usually in the younger age groups and have ulcers on the oral mucosa and gingivae, but suffer little systemic upset. There may be vesicles on the hands (and buttocks), and the parents should be asked to remove the child's shoes and socks to see if the feet are similarly affected.

Treatment

The disease is self-limiting, and again the treatment should be directed towards reassurance for the parents and maintenance of an adequate diet, including fluids. The contagious nature of the infection should be explained and the child should be reviewed in a week. Outbreaks of this disease are limited in extent and tend to occur in the summer months, but other children attending the practice or other family members may be affected.

Diagnosis

For confirmation of the diagnosis the virus may be isolated in the laboratory from vesicular fluid or throat swabs.

Epidemic parotitis

Epidemic parotitis is more commonly known as 'mumps', a term derived from an old English word 'mump', meaning to mope. It commonly infects children and adolescents between the ages of 5 and 15 years. The illness may start with general malaise, anorexia, headache and slight fever, although these symptoms are not always present. When salivary gland involvement occurs, it usually involves the parotid, and appears some 48 hours later.

Pain is located around the ear, together with swelling extending from the ear-lobe, which is everted over the angle of the mandible. It is extremely common for only one parotid to be involved; but even when both are affected they may not be so simultaneously. Indeed, swelling on the first side may have completely subsided before the contralateral side is affected.

Diagnosis

In view of the often unilateral presentation, confusion of the diagnosis with an acute alveolar abscess is not infrequent. Recurrent parotitis from other causes, such as glandular fever, should also be considered, particularly if the child has contacted someone with this condition.

Diagnosis can be confirmed by culture of the virus from saliva swabs or urine or by demonstration of a rising antibody titre.

Treatment

Pain is relieved by analgesics, oral cleanliness is maintained, and a liquid diet is provided if eating is difficult. Since complications are common and varied, the patient's general medical practitioner should be informed if she or he has not already been consulted.

Other conditions

Other viral and bacterial infections include varicella (chicken-pox), streptococcal sore throat and infectious mononucleosis (glandular fever), which are associated with oral vesicles (in the first case) and ulceration (in the second and third). Acute necrotizing ulcerative gingivitis in children is so rare now in the UK that if it is seen a problem with the child's underlying general health should be suspected. Note also that, though they are uncommon, oncology problems do arise in children, and the clinician should always be alert to this possibility, since it is crucial that the earliest referral possible is made.

Trauma

Introduction

Trauma is common in both the deciduous and the permanent dentition. The 1993 Children's Dental Health Survey recorded that a fifth of 13-year-olds surveyed had suffered dental trauma on at least one occasion. The only British National figures published relating specifically to deciduous incisors showed the prevalence in 5-year-olds to be 8 per cent, recorded by observation of discoloration, fracture, displacement or tooth loss. However it is generally accepted that trauma to primary incisors is commoner than this, occurring predominantly in the toddler age group (18 months to $2^1/_2$ years), when children are becoming more adventurous but are still unsteady on their feet.

The presentation can be upsetting, with an agitated parent arriving in the practice reception area with a young, distressed child in his or her arms. It is therefore imperative for the parent and the smooth running of the practice that these cases are seen immediately. Because trauma is likely to be associated with soft tissue injury, there may well be considerable bleeding. A small amount of blood appears much more when mixed with saliva, and, if smeared extra-orally, is disturbing to both parent and child. Washing the patient's face may achieve a dramatic improvement in appearances and in the reduction of stress levels.

Diagnosis

Although a full case history and examination are essential, only the most relevant details are necessary at first, viz how, when and where did the injury occur. A history of any previous dental trauma should be noted, and any noticeable difference in tooth position or disturbance of the occlusion should be recorded. A short medical history, identifying any serious conditions or allergies and tetanus status should be taken. Acquiring this information is often speeded up by asking the accompanying adult to complete a medical proforma whilst still in the reception area.

For future reference it is essential that a more detailed history is recorded accurately at a later stage. This would prove particularly helpful in the event of a request for a medico-legal report.

Clinical examination is undertaken after cleaning the patient's face with water or a mild antiseptic such as Savlon (Zeneca, UK). Soft tissue lacerations are examined, and, if a penetrating wound is detected, the presence of a foreign body, such as missing or fractured portions of teeth, as well as dirt, gravel or glass, should be considered. The teeth are dried and examined for fracture into enamel, dentine or pulp, and tested for mobility and displacement. Mobility should be tested by applying pressure labio-palatally, as well as in the long axis of the tooth. Any crevicular haemorrhage should be noted, as it may be indicative of luxation and/or root fracture. Vitality testing is unreliable in children, particularly following dental trauma, when concussion of the tooth may preclude positive response for up to six weeks.

Radiographs are taken where indicated and practicable. A soft tissue film may be necessary to locate foreign bodies if there is a deep lip laceration. This can be taken by placing a dental radiograph inside the lip and in front of the teeth and exposing for a quarter of the normal time. When, in the deciduous dentition, a view of the upper anterior teeth is necessary, an occlusal view using a small film (size 2) gives a satisfactory view of root and alveolar fractures as well as luxation injuries, and ascertains whether an intruded deciduous incisor has invaded the follicle of the permanent tooth germ.

In the very young child the possibility of non-accidental injury must be taken into account. If the injuries seen do not accord with those expected from the history, or if there is evidence of an unexpected unrelated injury or old bruising and physical abuse is suspected, the general practitioner or a hospital paediatrician should be contacted. Clearly, if the injury is more severe, immediate transfer to hospital is indicated.

Soft tissue injuries

Soft tissue injury is not usually severe; however a deep, gaping, extra-oral facial laceration may be treated with Steristrips (Ethicon, Edinburgh) or tissue glue, while a through-and-through lip laceration requires suturing. A 3/0 Vicryl suture (Ethicon, Edinburgh) should be used, which may either be removed in 7 days or be allowed to resorb over several weeks.

Abrasions containing grit or other foreign matter are not uncommon, and should be cleansed as soon as possible. This can be accomplished simply by washing with gauze or a sponge soaked in antiseptic. For the firmly attached but very localized particles light scrubbing under local anaesthesia using a toothbrush or other suitable instrument may be necessary, and larger particles may be picked out with a fine pair of tweezers. Where foreign bodies are deeply embedded or abrasions are extensive and particularly contaminated with debris and co-operation is failing, secondary referral to a hospital department might be appropriate, especially if general anaesthesia is likely to be required.

Injuries to the deciduous dentition

Luxation injuries, particularly intrusion, are the most frequent in this age group probably a result of the crown/root ratio and resilient alveolar bone. Fracture is rare, and when it occurs coronally, the crown of the tooth usually has a line of weakness – often a pre-existing carious lesion.

Management

This should be planned with the health of the permanent successor in mind. Thus, injuries displacing the primary incisor into the permanent tooth follicle should be treated by extraction. Infection at the site of trauma is common, owing either to plaque impaction – when infection occurs within a few days – or to infection of the necrotic pulp of the traumatized tooth – when infection occurs at a later date. The patient should be monitored at frequent intervals, and if either occurs the causative tooth should be extracted.

Crown fractures

Many consist simply of chipped enamel, in which case it should be possible to smooth the sharp edge. However, if there is considerable dentine or pulpal involvement, extraction may be the treatment of choice. Crown fracture is commonly associated with an underlying carious lesion. It is then useful to examine the first deciduous molars as well as the contra-lateral teeth to ascertain whether these also require treatment. Depending on the co-operation of the child and the choice of anaesthetic, treatment of all teeth may be expedited at the same time.

Root fractures

These are rare, but may be treated conservatively by advising a soft diet and review rather than attempting splinting – which is extremely difficult to accomplish in young children. Should infection follow, it is usually limited to the pulp of the coronal segment, and this portion of the tooth will then require extraction. The apical fragment can, and should, be left to resorb in the normal way.

Luxation

Luxation of primary teeth is by far the most common injury. The tooth is most frequently either undisplaced, intruded or the crown is retroclined. Consequently displacement is usually away from the developing tooth germ. Unless the displacement interferes with the occlusion, the luxated incisor can successfully be left untreated. If the incisor interferes with the occlusion and the child presents within a short period of time following the accident, the tooth can be manually repositioned using firm, steady and confident digital pressure. Local analgesia is seldom required.

Crown proclination should be treated with suspicion, because it is the type of luxation most likely to result in impaction of the root into the permanent tooth follicle. A radiograph is essential, and if the traumatized deciduous tooth appears elongated, this can be taken as confirmation. When the tooth is displaced in this way, extraction is advisable, and should be undertaken by application of forceps only (following appropriate analgesia), since the use of elevators may further damage the developing tooth germ. If it is impossible to hold the tooth in the normal labio-palatal direction, it may be possible to grasp it by placing the blades of the forceps mesio-distally.

Traumatic loss

Should a child have been unfortunate enough to exarticulate a deciduous tooth during the traumatic episode, replantation is contra-indicated. Unless the tooth can be produced for examination its apparent absence from the mouth should not be taken as sufficient evidence that it has been lost – it could be severely enough intruded to have disappeared from view. If a radiograph reveals the latter to be the case, the tooth should be allowed to re-erupt spontaneously while the situation is monitored by review appointments: initially at one week and subsequently at monthly intervals.

Follow-up

Following all forms of soft tissue or dental trauma, local cleansing measures and a soft diet are advised. Prescription of antibiotics is rarely necessary. Paracetamol is the analgesic of choice, while the need for its administration may be left to the discretion of the parent. If the wound is contaminated and the parents are uncertain of the anti-tetanus titre, they should be recommended to visit their GP for advice and/or treatment as appropriate. Arrangements should be made to review the patient in approximately one week. It is advisable to mention to parents the possibility of damage to the underlying permanent tooth, but not in such a way as to alarm them unduly. The timing of this information is important, and it is best imparted at the review appointment, when the parents will be more receptive to advice.

All traumatized patients should be monitored in both the short and long term, since pulpal necrosis may eventually occur in up to 50 per cent of teeth. Provided that the patient normally attends for routine care, this should be easily managed on a 4 or 6 month recall basis. Discoloration of traumatized deciduous teeth is frequent, but not necessarily indicative of non-vitality. Progressive yellowing of the tooth denotes calcification of the pulp chamber, while a consistent and continued darkening towards grey may indicate pulp necrosis. Early discoloration to grey (i.e. in the first month post-trauma) should be left to be reassessed. The tooth may remain vital and the discoloration may often lighten considerably, though not ultimately to its original colour.

It is particularly important to check for the normal and timely exfoliation of damaged teeth. Untreated non-vital teeth, though symptomless, may be surrounded apically by an area of sterile necrosis, which in turn may prevent physiological root resorption and lead to retention of the deciduous tooth. This can result in delayed eruption of the permanent successor or its deviation from the normal path of eruption. If permanent upper incisors become deflected palatally they may become trapped in reverse overjet, with the erupted lower incisors creating an orthodontic problem that will require appliance therapy later.

Injuries of the permanent dentition

In the permanent dentition, trauma most commonly results in crown fractures, which may or may not be associated with a luxation injury. Root fracture and exarticulation are relatively uncommon, but more difficult to treat, the latter requiring immediate attention.

Management

As in the younger age group, following trauma, the child and accompanying adult are both often extremely upset. Even for a child who attends regularly, this may be the first time for active dental treatment. Added to this there is the shock of dental injury in a patient who may not previously have experienced dental disease. In addition to the discomfort, soft tissue injury and temporary disfigurement may prove overwhelming. Although the patient's immediate concern may well be for appearance, the practitioner must concentrate initially on maintenance of pulp vitality and treatment of periodontal ligament damage.

Crown fractures

In the absence of a luxation injury, chipped enamel seldom requires immediate treatment. At a later visit sharp or rough edges may be smoothed or the missing portion replaced with acid-etch composite.

A fracture through enamel and dentine necessitates immediate treatment to seal the dentinal tubules and protect the underlying pulp. Treatment to restore the appearance is less urgent, and can be delayed to a later visit. Sealing of the exposed dentinal tubules is achieved using hard-setting calcium hydroxide, glass–ionomer cement or a dentine-bonding agent, of which hard-setting calcium hydroxide is most popular. On no account should a zinc oxide/eugenol-containing cement be used if the ultimate restoration will be a composite resin build-up, since eugenol interferes with resin polymerization.

The limitation of hard-setting calcium hydroxide is that it is easily dislodged, and must therefore be held in place. This can be accomplished by the use of the crown fragment itself, a composite resin 'bandage', a temporary crown of composite, acrylic or stainless steel, or an orthodontic band. Whichever method is used, the whole of the exposed dentinal surface is first covered with the calcium hydroxide. Where sufficient enamel remains, the simplest method is then to etch the palatal and labial enamel and, after washing and drying, cover it with unfilled composite resin. This technique is relatively simple even for an anxious patient with soft tissue swelling or laceration. If the tooth fragment is available, this may still be utilized at a later date, although in the interim it should be stored in isotonic saline. The use of a temporary crown may be necessary where the tooth has insufficient supragingival enamel for retention. This is unusual in an enamel/dentine fracture without luxation, but may be necessary when the fracture involves the pulp.

The tooth must be considered to be exposed when the dentine is so thin that the pulp shadow is visible even if there is no detectable perforation. Treatment then depends on the time interval before presentation and the stage of tooth development. If pulp vitality is to be maintained pulp capping or even partial pulpotomy are the treatments of choice rather than full coronal pulpotomy. Pulp capping is most successful on 'near' or very small exposures seen within 24 hours of injury. After isolation of the tooth, a layer of hard-setting calcium hydroxide dressing is applied and sealed tightly in place with an acid-etch composite or temporary crown.

For larger exposures or others which have occurred recently but more than 24 hours ago, partial pulpotomy is the treatment of choice. First local analgesia is administered. It may be necessary to supplement a buccal infiltration on both sides of the midline with a palatal infiltration or intraligamentary injection. Subsequently isolation is best achieved by placement of a rubber dam, although cotton wool rolls and a salivary ejector must suffice if this proves impossible. Access through the exposure is gained using a water-cooled high-speed handpiece fitted with a pear-shaped or inverted cone diamond bur. The underlying pulp tissue is removed to a depth of approximately 2 mm or until found to be bleeding normally, whichever is the sooner. The resultant haemorrhage should be controlled and arrested with cotton wool pledgets, subsequently to which a layer of calcium hydroxide – either in pure or hard-set form – should be used to cover the pulp. The cavity is sealed with glass–ionomer cement or composite resin prior to a temporary restoration.

The former recommendations have assumed the anterior tooth to be immature, and indeed this is likely in a patient of less than 15 years of age. However, should the tooth be mature, with a closed apex, small exposures seen within hours of the accident may be treated by pulp capping as described previously. Larger or older exposures should be treated by conventional endodontic techniques.

Follow-up

If at the initial visit a temporary restoration was not placed, either because of lack of patient co-operation or in the presence of substantial soft tissue injury, a subsequent visit within a short time-interval is essential. Where a contact point has been lost, adjacent teeth must be prevented from drifting into the available space. This is especially important in the crowded arch or at the time of eruption of the upper canine teeth. Thereafter traumatized teeth should be regularly monitored at approximately three-monthly intervals for a period of at least two years.

Root fractures

Fortunately root fracture is a relatively uncommon injury in children. It usually affects mature teeth with closed apices, and the patient is often a teenager or older. The affected tooth is usually mobile, but may not be displaced. Radiographic confirmation is often difficult, because the fracture line tends to run obliquely. It is advisable to take at least two periapical radiographs at different angulations in order to confirm the diagnosis and locate the fracture.

If displaced, the coronal fragment should be re-positioned by application of firm pressure to the tooth after disimpaction from any bony obstruction. Local analgesia is advisable. A successful approximation of the root fragments can often be judged clinically, but should also be confirmed by a further radiograph. The coronal fragment should then be maintained in this position by splinting for a period of three months. Acid-etch composite provides a most acceptable and convenient method of splinting. When extra stability and strength are required an orthodontic wire may be incorporated under the composite, but it is essential that this wire is passive. For such splinting to be successful it is also important that at least one tooth on either side of the fractured tooth is incorporated in order to act as an abutment.

Textbooks usually divide root fractures into apical, middle and gingival thirds. However, since the ultimate hope is for repair of the fracture, the immediate treatment is the same wherever the fracture line lies, unless it runs vertically, in which case extraction is necessary.

Table 6.1 Follow-up of trauma in the permanent dentition (based on Andreason and Andreason)

	Type of trauma			
	Root fracture	*Extrusion*	*Lateral luxation*	*Replantation*
1 week				Splint removal and endo. if apex closed
2–3 weeks	Radiograph	Radiograph and splint removal. Endo. if apex closed		Radiograph
6–8 weeks	Radiograph		Splint removal. Endo. if apex closed	Radiograph
3 months	Radiograph and splint removal			Radiograph
6 months				Radiograph
1 year	Radiograph		Radiograph	Radiograph
2–4 years				Radiograph
5, 10, 15 yrs	Radiograph	Radiograph	Radiograph	Radiograph

Follow-up

After-care is summarized in Table 6.1. The patient is instructed to make an earlier visit if any symptoms occur. Increased radiolucency at the fracture line caused by resorption of bone at the apical end of the coronal fragment is indicative of necrosis, and, if observed, is treated immediately by extirpation of the pulp down to the fracture line. The tooth is dressed with non-setting calcium hydroxide, and follow-up is as for open-apex, non-vital root canal treatment.

Should there be insufficient remaining crown to support a restoration, there may be indications for retaining the fragment and thereby maintaining the overlying supporting alveolar bone. Space is maintained by fitting a T-shaped partial denture. Alternatively both fragments may be removed and a partial denture may be fitted while healing takes place. In the long term an etch-bonded bridge or osseointegrated implant may be indicated.

Luxation injuries

Direct trauma to teeth may damage the periodontal ligament. In mild cases the teeth remain undisplaced although slightly mobile, with only crevicular haemorrhage visible. In others the teeth may be displaced laterally, intruded or extruded, and treatment is directed towards repositioning and splinting.

Teeth displaced laterally or extruded can be re-positioned by firm digital pressure. In the former case, local analgesia may be necessary, but is not usually required in the latter. The re-positioned teeth should be splinted for 2 to 3 weeks. The use of a methacrylate resin (e.g. Pro-temp, ESPE, Seefeld, Germany) following acid etching is recommended, since it is easier to remove than conventional composite. Mildly intruded teeth may re-erupt spontaneously if left. This is most likely when the tooth is immature, with a wide-open apex. In the early mixed dentition it may be difficult to judge the degree of intrusion because the level of eruption of the contralateral teeth is not necessarily symmetrical. Should the tooth fail to re-erupt spontaneously it may be gently extruded orthodontically, thereby minimizing further insult to the pulp. Where teeth have been severely intruded, they may have to be surgically re-positioned with forceps and splinted. The protocol for follow-up is shown in Table 6.1.

Tooth loss

This form of injury is relatively uncommon following trauma, but is more likely in 7- to 10-year-olds. It is often associated with soft tissue injury or fracture of the alveolar plate. The first contact may be a telephone call from the child's parent or teacher for advice and help. Where there are other injuries it is unlikely dental treatment will be the first priority for a caller. Nevertheless, it is worth enquiring whether the patient has lost consciousness; in which case a medical opinion is indicated. It is also worth confirming with the caller whether a permanent tooth is involved, either by establishing the age of the patient or by checking with dental records. Should this prove to be the case, it is most important to allay any fears and check if the tooth has indeed been knocked out, and if so, to locate it.

It is important to know the nature of the surface on to which the tooth has fallen and therefore judge the degree of contamination. If dirty, the tooth must be rinsed or sucked clean. If the patient/adult is then able to distinguish between labial and palatal surfaces, advice should be given on how to hold the tooth by the crown and replace it in the socket. If this proves too difficult, the child should be brought to the surgery, with the tooth, as quickly as possible. It can be transported either in the child's or parent's mouth, with the attendant potential risk of being swallowed, or in milk. The need for speed cannot be overemphasized, because the best prognosis for replantation occurs when the tooth is replaced within 30 minutes. Enquire how far away the patient is and the intended mode of travel to the surgery. It may be necessary to alert an alternative treatment centre nearer the scene of the accident and direct the patient there. On arrival at the practice the time elapsed is crucial, and the patient must not be kept waiting. Staff should be aware of the speed necessary when dealing with exarticulations, lest precious time is lost with the patient sat in a waiting-room!

On arrival, take a brief history of the accident, including the approximate time of injury and therefore the time lapse to the present, and establish the conditions under which the tooth has been stored. The exarticulated tooth is examined for obvious signs of contamination, as well as for caries, restorations, previous fracture or hypoplasia, before being placed in isotonic saline. A brief medical history is taken and checked to ensure that replantation is in the patient's best overall health interest.

Before making the decision to replant a tooth, examine the tooth socket and mouth as a whole. Although an extra-oral period of less than 30 minutes has been shown to give the best prognosis, and while one exceeding 2 hours is less successful, storage conditions are also important. While a tooth transported dry can usually be successfully replanted within a period of 30 min, a slightly longer extra-oral period of storage is possible when the tooth has been transported in saliva or milk.

Although the alveolar socket needs to be relatively intact to provide a good base for the replantation, time is of the essence, and pre-treatment radiographs should only be taken if there is a definite possibility of bony fracture. Provided the rest of the dentition is intact and the state of the tooth is aesthetically acceptable, it should be replanted as quickly as possible.

Since any interference with the root surface has a profound influence on healing, every care must be taken to handle the tooth by the crown alone. It is helpful to record the state of root development and to measure the length of the tooth – if root canal treatment becomes necessary, this useful observation may save a diagnostic X-ray. It is now thought beneficial to wash the socket with saline in order to remove clot, as well as gently rinsing the root surface with saline to remove bacteria. The tooth can be replanted using digital pressure. It is likely that the tooth will be immature, with a short straight root, and therefore little resistance will be met. If, however, the socket wall is fractured, local analgesia may be needed, and the socket wall can be remodelled with a Couplands elevator. After replacing the tooth, it should be held in place with a splint.

For many years a suck-down splint with total upper-arch coronal coverage was preferred by those dentists with rapid access to a laboratory. Co-operation was facilitated by the use of a lower tray (so avoiding palatal coverage) after applying Vaseline to the replanted tooth. If necessary mild intrusion of the replanted tooth could be effected by trimming the incisal edge on the model. More recent practice, now preferred where there are sound teeth alongside, is to acid etch-bond the reimplanted tooth to an adjacent abutment. This has the advantage that the palatal surface remains uncovered, facilitating access should root canal treatment be required. In the event that suitable adjacent teeth are available, an acid-etch-retained splint should be applied for 7–10 days.

A five-day course of antibiotic therapy should be prescribed immediately, and the patient should be referred to his or her general medical practitioner with a report of the accident for advice regarding tetanus immunization.

Follow-up

Appointments for follow-up should be made as recommended in Table 6.1. Should there be radiographic evidence of periapical radiolucency or surface resorption of the root – the latter being indicated by a moth-eaten appearance – then necrotic pulp tissue should be extirpated and the canal should be dressed with non-setting calcium hydroxide. The necessity to undertake this with some urgency cannot be overemphasized, since inflammatory resorption once started can progress extremely rapidly, with resultant destruction of the root. Pulp extirpation followed by dressing with alkaline bactericidal calcium hydroxide halts the process. This should then be followed in the same way as for a non-vital, open-apex root canal treatment.

Orthodontic appliances

Patients undergoing active orthodontic treatment can experience acute problems with both fixed and removable appliances. Although treatment may sometimes be supervised by an orthodontist, quite frequently the patient will need help from his local or 'on call' dental practitioner. The most common dental emergencies related to fixed appliances occur when components become loose or are embedded in soft tissue. Emergencies with removable appliances tend to be fracture of the acrylic base plate or retaining cribs or distortion of other metal components.

Fixed appliances

Generalized discomfort is frequently associated with a newly fitted arch wire. When this occurs, the patient should keep to a soft diet and analgesics should be recommended for 48 hours if necessary. The patient should be advised to contact the supervising practitioner if the symptoms persist beyond 2 days.

Localized pain most frequently occurs in relation to a banded molar tooth. Where there is associated swelling, it is imperative to check whether the band is loose, in which case its removal should provide relief. It may prove necessary to cut the arch wire in front of the affected tooth in order to allow band removal. Once free, the tooth should be cleaned both supra- and subgingivally to remove all cement and plaque. Depending on the degree of swelling, antibiotics may be necessary, and the patient should be instructed to contact her or his orthodontist as soon as possible. The band should be placed in a suitable container and returned to the patient to present to the orthodontist at that visit.

Where the end of an arch wire impacts into the cheek there will be obvious soft tissue irritation in relation to a molar tooth. If sufficient arch wire is visible, it should be bent into a more comfortable position. Should a significant amount still protrude, it can be cut off after bending down the end. Wax or a similar material may then be placed over the end of the offending wire to prevent further soft tissue trauma.

Brackets, loops, hooks and buccal tubes can also cause soft tissue irritation. Red carding wax provided by the orthodontist, or chewing gum or Blu-tac supplied by the patient, are some of the materials more commonly used to cover sharp extensions. Clear utility wax may also be used, and has a less dramatic appearance – the patient does not look as if he or she is eating a cherry! Most recently clear silicone (Brace Gard, Infa-Labtic, Rockaway, NJ) has been marketed, and, since it requires less pressure to apply, this is particularly helpful when the teeth carrying the wire components are mobile or tender.

Before applying silicone or wax, the relevant area should be dried with tissue or gauze. Sufficient material is then applied and can be moulded with pressure from a wet finger, using a fingernail to push it over and round the tube or bracket and achieve retention. As a palliative measure, an antiseptic gel (e.g. Brace Relief, Infa-Labtic, Rockaway, NJ) can be recommended. These materials are particularly helpful when the soft tissues covering anterior brackets become sore, as is often the case with wind instrument players.

Removable appliances

The major causes of soft tissue ulceration are usually the buccal springs or labial bows on simple removable appliances or lingual extensions on functional appliances. Should soft tissue inflammation or ulceration be caused by acrylic, this may be trimmed in the same way as easing a denture. If the 'wire work' is causing a problem this may be recontoured. Should this fail to produce a significant improvement the patient should, as a last resort, be asked to leave the appliance out. When this occurs it is important to emphasize the necessity to visit the orthodontist as soon as possible, so that corrective treatment may recommence with the minimum of delay.

When a patient presents with an acrylic fracture where only a small portion has been lost, it may be sufficient to trim the sharp edges. However, if there is a significant fracture of the appliance and the original working model is unavailable, it will be necessary to take an impression and return the plate to the laboratory for repair. This impression is preferably taken with the appliance in the mouth; but depending on the position or extent of the fracture an impression may be taken without the appliance, provided that it can be easily located on the resulting model. Similarly, if an active or passive metal component or crib is fractured, it should be repaired by soldering as soon as possible. If a new crib is required, an impression with the appliance in place will almost certainly be necessary. Where other wires have been broken they should first be made safe by removing sharp ends.

Occasionally a problem arises when a patient is unable to insert or remove an appliance. To avoid this situation both patient and parent should be familiar with the fitting and removing techniques before leaving the surgery, and have demonstrated their ability to remove and reinsert the appliance with all its components in the correct position.

Headgear

Both fixed and removable appliances may be supported by headgear. In the event of severe discomfort, the patient should temporarily cease wear and be advised to return to the orthodontist as soon as possible. Patients and their parents must be warned against the dangers of attempting to adjust the appliance themselves. Penetrating wounds of eye and skin have been caused by the misuse of self-adjusted headgear.

Table 6.2 National Poisons Information Service – 24 hr emergency telephone numbers

London	0171 635 9191
Edinburgh	0131 229 2477
Cardiff	01222 709901
Belfast	01232 240503
Dublin	0001 379966
Regional service available in:	
Birmingham	0121 554 3801
Newcastle	0191 232 5131

Fluoride intoxication

The use of fluoride both systemically and topically in a variety of products has proved most effective in reducing dental caries in the young patient. Although such fluoride products are generally very safe, it is still imperative to exercise caution in their use. The dental surgeon should be fully aware of the potential dangers of over-dosage. In addition he should be in a position to advise on appropriate treatment should over-dosage occur.

Fortunately incidents of lethal intoxication with fluoride are rare. The majority relate to suicides, but a number occur accidentally. In 1943, 47 patients died in a single incident in the US as a direct result of sodium fluoride powder being mistaken for sodium chloride and added to food.

In this country reports of drug over-dosage are monitored by the National Poisons Information Service (Table 6.2). This is conducted in a similar manner to the monitoring of adverse drug reactions by the Committee on Safety of Medicines. Medical and dental practitioners are encouraged to report unusual or severe cases to the service. This information service is responsible for identifying the level of a lethal dose of fluoride in the United Kingdom, the figure being quoted in relation to body weight. The lower limit is thought to be approximately 30 mg of elemental fluoride per kilogram body weight. This is equivalent to 2.5 gm of fluoride ion for the average adult male. Fluoride is most commonly encountered in the form of sodium fluoride, every 2.2 gm of which contain 1 gm of fluoride ion. From these figures, an adult male who ingests 5 gm of sodium fluoride would receive a certainly lethal dose (CLD).

To date there have only been three fatal cases of fluoride intoxication by ingestion of dental products in young children aged between 2 and 3 years. In one case it was evident that a dose of only 5 mg per kilogram was responsible; therefore a quantity as small as this should be regarded as potentially lethal. The amount of fluoride which can produce acute poisoning is considerably less; it is variously quoted as being between 1 mg and 20 mg of sodium fluoride per kilogram. In the average adult male, toxic symptoms may therefore become evident after ingestion of as little as 70 mg of fluoride or 150 mg of sodium fluoride. When these ratios are applied to children, who are considerably lighter, it is evident that only a very small amount need be ingested before symptoms may become apparent. Consequently acute fluoride poisoning may be possible either from careless application of high-fluoride-concentration products in the dental surgery, or through misuse of commercially available preparations in the home.

Acute intoxication

Early symptoms of fluoride poisoning occur within 30–60 minutes of ingestion. Should fluoride have been ingested in the dental surgery in sufficient quantity to cause symptoms, the patient is likely to have left the surgery and to be travelling or to have returned home. Symptoms of fluoride intoxication include nausea, vomiting, hypersalivation, abdominal pain and diarrhoea. It is worth noting that, depending on the mode of transport home, these symptoms in a child might also be inadvertently attributed to car sickness. Where a considerable quantity of fluoride has been ingested, muscular weakness, spasms and tetany may follow, and in the few cases of fatal poisoning which have been reported, death usually occurred within 24 hours as a result of respiratory or cardiac failure.

In any case of suspected fluoride poisoning, three items of information are essential, namely the exact fluoride preparation, the quantity swallowed and the weight of the patient. Table 6.3 lists the procedure to follow if fluoride poisoning is suspected.

Chronic fluoride intoxication

In areas where the natural level of fluoride in the water is less than optimal, a child may receive fluoride supplementation in the form of tablets or drops. These can be prescribed by the dentist or purchased over the counter by the parent. Frequently the clinician is asked to advise on a child's taking fluoride supplementation when spending time away from home. The time-interval involved may be a short vacation or a more prolonged period. In either case it is recommended to ascertain the level of fluoride in the water supply of the neighbourhood that the child will be visiting.

Table 6.3 Emergency procedures to follow in cases of suspected fluoride poisoning

Fluoride ion ingested per kg body weight	*Treatment*
<5	Drink a large volume of milk in order to slow the absorption of the fluoride.
5–15	Drink large amounts of milk on the way to hospital, where an emetic mixture will be given (e.g. Paediatric BP Ipecac. Syrup) to empty the stomach. Milk, Epsom salts or aluminium hydroxide antacid mixture should then be taken to slow absorption of any remaining fluoride.
>15	Immediate transfer to hospital for gastric lavage.

In Britain this information can be obtained by contacting the regional water board or the nearest Consultant in Dental Public Health. If the child is planning a trip abroad, where the water fluoride level is uncertain, it is generally advisable to recommend that systemic fluoride is discontinued for the duration of the stay. This advice is also applicable for travel to a country in which bottled water is used, since the fluoride levels contained in such water may be high. Plasma fluoride levels are rapidly affected by alteration in fluoride intake, and thus, if raised above the optimal level, enamel formation may be disturbed, and, even though there is a relatively short period of chronic intoxication, this may be sufficient to lead to mild mottling of the teeth.

Previous assumptions on the prescription of fluoride supplementation have been based on a belief that the general public drinks tap water. However, sales of bottled waters have tripled in recent years. These waters may not be bottled in the immediate locality, and those readily available in supermarkets in the UK contain between 0.01 and 1.0 ppm of fluoride. Fortunately, all bottled water now has to have the fluoride content shown on the label, and this should be checked before purchase when living in a fluoridated area. It may therefore be worth checking with a parent as to the nature and quantity of the normal fluid intake of the household prior to any consideration of fluoride supplementation.

7

Post-operative problems

Keith Figures

Local conditions affecting hard tissue

Enamel is a tissue which undergoes no biological change with age, but does suffer from structural change with age. Changes include the development of enamel cracks, which occur more commonly in heavily restored teeth that experience excessive occlusal load. The presence of enamel cracks may allow the tooth structure to flex, particularly if a cusp is affected. This can give rise to discomfort during function: hence the term 'cracked tooth syndrome', which is discussed in Chapter 2.

Dentine is a dynamic tissue, which, unlike enamel, undergoes continual change throughout life. Increased mineralization occurs, and can be seen in older teeth as translucent root dentine, particularly around the apex of the tooth. The colour of dentine may change to a deeper yellow or brown in older teeth, especially if the dentine has been exposed to the oral environment. In addition, a reduction in pulp size will occur, owing to the deposition of secondary dentine, resulting in an apical migration of the coronal pulp and a coronal migration of the apical constriction. This may complicate or contra-indicate endodontic treatment.

Cementum, like dentine, is a dynamic tissue undergoing continual deposition throughout life, and as a result the root length can increase. When the effects of secondary dentine formation and cementum deposition are combined the relationship of the apical root constriction to the radiographic root apex changes, and this should be borne in mind when performing endodontic therapy on the older patient.

Tooth wear

Tooth wear is the loss of mineralized tooth tissue as a result of physical and/or chemical attack. It is a natural phenomenon, and to a degree occurs with increasing age. However, in some individuals tooth wear is excessive, and may be considered pathological.

Three forms of tooth wear are recognized:

- **Attrition.** This results from tooth-to-tooth contact and may be seen in bruxism.
- **Abrasion.** This is due to tooth tissue loss caused by factors other than mastication or bruxing, and a good example is toothbrush abrasion due to an inappropriate toothbrushing technique.
- **Erosion.** Chemical agents (not from plaque) are responsible for this form of tooth substance loss.

Attrition

The extent to which attrition occurs is dependent on the use to which individuals put their teeth. In some groups where the diet is abrasive the degree of attrition is high. For example, desert-dwelling people such as the Bedouin demonstrate high levels of attrition due to the sand they ingest with their food. However, in the UK the commonest reasons for attrition are the loss of posterior teeth, forcing more chewing to be done on anterior teeth, which are poorly adapted to this role and so wear down quickly. Secondly, parafunctional habits that involve the performance of abnormal grinding or clenching movements can be very destructive to tooth substance.

The aetiology of parafunction can be complex, but emotional, psychological, systemic, occupational and of course idiopathic factors must be investigated. Systemic problems arise in patients with dyskynesias in which involuntary jaw movement may be seen, as in some elderly patients. This picture can be complicated if there is an additional erosive element that is contributing to the tooth-substance loss. When this happens the exposed dentine will be removed more quickly than the surrounding enamel, so producing 'dishing' of the contact surfaces, as in Figure 7.1.

Abrasion

There are two types of wear categorized as abrasion. The first is seen in individuals who work in a dusty atmosphere, such as coal mines or cutlery manufacturers, and who ignore the Health and Safety at Work regulations by not wearing facial masks. Tiny particles of grit adhere to the teeth, and act as a grinding paste when combined with saliva. This type of abrasion is less common now as a result of better working conditions, but nevertheless is still occasionally seen.

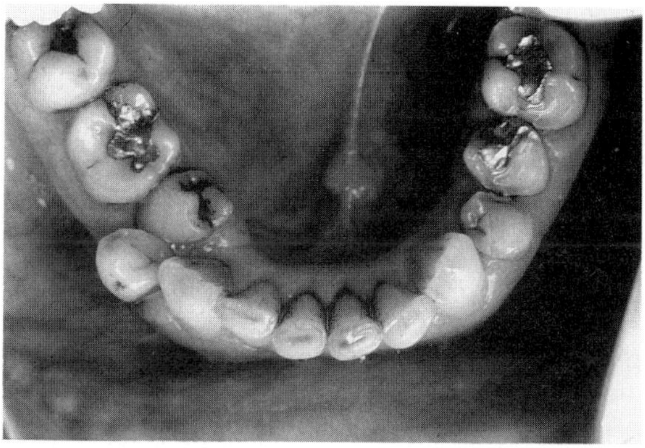

Figure 7.1 Tooth surfaces demonstrating attrition exacerbated by erosion.

Secondly and more commonly, abrasion is seen as a result of the use or abuse of oral hygiene aids such as toothbrushes, dental floss and other interdental aids like bottle brushes. Over-zealous scaling and polishing will also remove tooth substance, and it has been estimated that polishing teeth with an ordinary prophylactic paste will remove up to 4 μm of enamel each time teeth are polished. Abrasion due to using a stain-removing dentifrice such as smoker's tooth powder can cause significant abrasion, and this type of oral hygiene product is to be discouraged.

Erosion

This is quite commonly seen now in young adults who have less than ideal dietary habits. The easy availability of carbonated soft drinks and lager beers with a low pH is partly to blame. In addition, the incidence of bulimia, where acidic stomach contents are regurgitated, will produce erosion in the young, while dyspepsia may explain erosion in the older patient. The alcoholic patient who vomits regularly can demonstrate erosion, and this may be the first indication of alcohol abuse in middle-class patients who are unwilling to admit their addiction. A careful history is required in cases of suspected erosion, and a diet-diary should be completed.

The typical pattern of tooth surface loss seen in this type of tooth wear is shown in Figure 7.1.

Management

When abnormal tooth wear is detected it is important initially to monitor this by using serial study models or clinical photographs.

If the wear is perceived to be progressing, or a stage has been reached where any further loss would make restorative reconstruction difficult, then restoration of the worn dentition should be considered. This will involve careful treatment-planning, starting with prevention and, if possible, elimination of any aetiological factors.

Prevention

There are a number of steps that can be taken to prevent tooth wear getting worse. In the case of erosion, dietary counselling is essential to identify acidic components of the diet. Conversely, in the case of a patient with achlorhydria, where normal gastric acid secretion is depleted, dilute hydrochloric acid may be being taken by mouth. In such a case it is helpful to advise the patient to take the medication into the mouth using a straw, to minimize tooth-surface contact. It is also helpful in these cases, where medication is thought to be responsible for the erosion, to contact the patient's medical practitioner and inform her or him of the problem, so that a different preparation or drug (if available) may be considered.

When the erosion is the result of acid regurgitation, prevention is more difficult. Patients suspected of suffering from anorexia nervosa with bulimia, or chronic alcoholism with vomiting, should be referred to a physician or psychiatrist for additional help. In those who are taking medication which, as a side-effect, induces nausea or vomiting, the help of the patient's physician should be sought. Even some diabetics are prone to this type of regurgitation erosion, and this should be borne in mind.

If times can be identified when the erosion is most likely to occur then it may be useful to construct a soft vinyl guard to wear at this time. Some authorities advise the placing of a fluoride gel or an antacid inside the guard before use. In addition, there is evidence that topical fluoride therapy is beneficial to patients at risk of erosive tooth-substance loss, and some advocate a similar management routine to that used for those with xerostomia. When the erosion is due to an adverse industrial environment then appropriate measures to protect the mouth from acid vapour should be instituted by both the patient and the company.

Attrition prevention

Wear as a result of normal chewing cannot be prevented; in fact some believe that this type of wear will increase in proportion to the amount of fibre present in the diet. The pattern of wear seen in Third World nationals is also common in those from the ethnic minorities in Western countries. In these patients the difficulty is to decide if treatment is either needed or wanted.

In the case of a bruxing habit management includes the provision of either a soft or hard occlusal guard, with or without occlusal adjustment, psychological counselling and in some cases psychotropic medication. Generally, however, guards are considered to be beneficial to the extent that they allow wear to occur on the appliance rather than the teeth.

It is especially important to be aware of bruxing before embarking on extensive restorative care. This is particularly true if porcelain is being used in the reconstruction. The reason is that the hardness of porcelain – particularly if poorly glazed or if eased in the surgery – will present a rough surface, and rapidly wear the opposing tooth. Therefore it is always preferable to have natural teeth contacting a metal surface, or, if this impossible, a highly glazed porcelain surface.

Abrasion prevention

It is important to identify the source of the damage first. If the working environment is dusty then the use of a face mask is essential. By teaching correct oral hygiene techniques and discouraging use of the teeth to hold objects such as pens, darning needles, etc. this type of wear can be controlled.

Soft tissue damage

Patients are very aware of the delicate nature of the soft tissues in the mouth, and one of their concerns about undergoing dental treatment is that these tissues will become traumatized. Clinicians must always be careful when dealing with soft tissues, taking care to use suitable finger rests when using rotating instruments, and non-reflecting or blackened retractors when using a laser. The gingivae are often mildly traumatized during many restorative procedures, but with care this can be kept to a minimum. The anxious patient may flinch unexpectedly during use of the high-speed handpiece, and both the assistant and the clinician should be prepared for this by making sure the soft tissues are retracted effectively and protected adequately.

Some patients who have a very strong and active tongue can be difficult to treat. It may then help to retract the tongue with an oral surgery tongue retractor held by the assistant, which will not only control the tongue but also provide protection for the tongue from the bur. The assistant's other hand can then hold the high-volume suction, which can also control tongue movement. The use of a rubber dam may also be indicated.

When patients have had a dental local analgesic they should always be warned of the possibility of trauma to the lip while anaesthesia persists. This is particularly true for children and mentally compromised patients. In addition, the medical defence societies advise that patients should be warned that lip sensation will be abnormal for the next hour or two.

The dentist is also responsible for the actions of the assistant, who, particularly if inexperienced, should be warned of the possibility of damage to alveolar mucosa or the floor of the mouth during aspiration. Metal aspirating tips are especially liable to inflict this, and the patient will not become aware of it until the local anaesthetic has worn off. When an injury of this type occurs inform the patient, and if necessary close the wound with a suture.

On occasions a soft tissue injury occurs which involves skin or other extra-oral structures such as the eyes. It is most important to deal with this type of injury effectively. The wearing of protective spectacles by all present will help reduce eye injury; but if it does occur then an ophthalmic opinion must be sought from the nearest hospital department. A telephone call to the local consultant ophthalmic surgeon for initial advice is recommended. When a facial injury has occurred the worry is that a permanent scar may result. This type of injury can occur when a hand instrument such as a scaler suddenly breaks, and the skin around the mouth is lacerated as a consequence. In this instance the laceration must be cleaned with an antiseptic solution such as cetrimide to remove any debris, and a decision must be made on whether suturing is required. A simple scratch may be covered with a butterfly-type dressing, but if the injury is deeper then the use of a very fine suture such as 6.0 Ethylon® is recommended. This is likely to require a referral to the local hospital accident and emergency department, and a telephone call to let them know the patient is coming is helpful. Ultimately, if a scar results, the opinion of a plastic surgeon may be sought by the patient. This may have medico-legal implications, and advice from your defence society would be prudent.

Care should also be taken when using chemicals or medicaments in or around the mouth which, if spilt, might burn skin or damage clothing. Careless use of acid etchants or root canal medicaments may cause these problems, and for this reason they should never be handed by the dental nurse to the dentist over the patient's face. If such a liquid is dropped on to the patient wash it off with copious amounts of water. As patients are now routinely treated in the supine position this type of incident is more common, and a lapse of concentration is all that it takes.

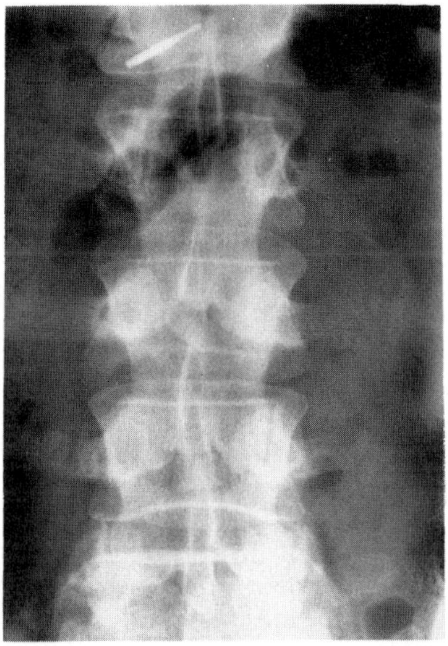

Figure 7.2 This finishing bur was not secured in the handpiece correctly, resulting in its being swallowed. It could just as easily have been inhaled, as the clinician had momentarily lost concentration.

Inhalation of a foreign body

As dentistry involves working in the mouth, often with quite tiny implements, it is to the credit of the dentist and the patients' protective reflexes that inhalation happens so infrequently. Nevertheless, it can occur quite easily and unexpectedly, particularly when the patient is supine. It usually occurs when the clinician has a momentary loss of concentration, for example not placing a bur correctly in the handpiece, as shown in Figure 7.2, or when the patient moves unexpectedly. In some patients it is important to be aware that they are at risk of inhaling a foreign body because their sensation to the throat may be impaired, as can occur in some patients with multiple sclerosis. For this reason or if the cough reflex is defective then it is advisable not to treat the patient in the supine position.

When a foreign body disappears the first stage is to see if it is lying elsewhere in the mouth. If a bur breaks unexpectedly it may still be in the operative site or may have been aspirated by high-volume suction, particularly if the patient has not suddenly swallowed or started coughing. If the foreign body cannot be found an explanation to the patient is essential, and a telephone call to the local consultant radiologist to explain what has happened and to seek his advice is recommended. Arrangements can then be made for the patient to be seen immediately and for the appropriate investigations to be undertaken. If the object is not visible on a chest film (assuming it is radiopaque) then it has probably been swallowed, and it will pass out naturally in a day or so without further treatment. Radiologists do not routinely take abdominal films to identify foreign bodies in the GI tract, as this is now considered to be an unnecessary radiation exposure. When the chest film reveals that inhalation has occurred it may be prudent to inform your defence society and seek their advice regarding the medico-legal implications.

Instrument loss

Occasionally a hand instrument tip is lost. An example would be fracture of a scaling instrument while scaling or root planing. It is most important to locate the mislaid piece, as it will, in all probability, be somewhere in the patient's mouth. Fracture is most likely to occur with instruments which are old or poorly maintained. Scaling instruments must be sharpened regularly to preserve their efficiency, and it is useful to remember that a sharp instrument will require less effort to remove calculus than a blunt one and therefore should be less likely to break. Ideally scaling instruments should be sharpened every week to preserve their efficiency. An assistant can undertake this function after being properly instructed.

Rarely, a brand new instrument may break. The fragments should be sent for metallurgical analysis, to prove the instrument was faulty at the time of manufacture. When a new instrument does break it should always be returned to the manufacturer in case there is a design fault – it will usually be replaced free of charge. High-speed burs can break when in use, and the fragment is usually aspirated, particularly if high volume suction is being used. Again a search of the mouth for the fragment should be undertaken, just in case it has not been aspirated. Particular attention should be paid to the posterior aspect of the dorsum of the tongue. Instrument loss may also occur during endodontics, a subject covered in Chapter 4 and needing no further comment here.

Needle fracture and needle track infection

Fortunately needle fracture is rare in clinical practice, owing to the universal use of disposable needles. Nevertheless, the clinician must be prepared for the eventuality of needle fracture, because quick retrieval of the fragment from the soft tissues is essential, as the broken fragment will submerge quickly. Once it has submerged it can be very difficult to locate surgically, and for this reason all dental students are advised never to insert a needle as far as the hub. The needle is more likely to fracture at the hub, and so long as a portion of the needle projects from the site it can be grasped with a pair of artery forceps and quickly removed. For this reason it is advisable to always have a pair of artery forceps readily accessible in the dental surgery.

Another advantage of using pre-sterilized disposable needles is the dramatic reduction in the incidence of needle track infection. True needle track infection is extremely rare today, but when an injection such as an inferior alveolar block or a posterior superior dental block is planned, then it should be delayed if there is inflammation in the area through which the needle will pass. It may be sensible to control the infection giving rise to the inflammation by means of antibiotics before administering the LA, in order to avoid spreading infection into the pterygo-mandibular space or the infratemporal fossa. Infections of the infratemporal fossa will make the patient very ill. Temperatures of 40° C are possible, and intracranial spread to the cavernous sinus a distinct possibility.

Occasionally, limitation of opening occurs after an inferior alveolar block, and this becomes progressively worse over the following days. This can be very painful, particularly if the patient tries to open the mandible past the point of limitation. This is probably due to bruising in the medial pterygoid muscle, and residual limitation of opening can be treated by using increasing numbers of tongue spatulas between the front teeth – slowly stretching the bruised muscle. It may be appropriate in such cases to refer to a physiotherapist in order to restore correct function, and this type of treatment is now becoming more popular. Some pain in the injection site after anaesthesia has worn off is not uncommon, but can be minimized by a careful and unrushed technique.

Accidental cross-infection

Accidents do occur in the clinical environment, but good surgery cross-infection control procedures should minimize their incidence. Such procedures should include the regular use of needle guards like Aim-Safe (Septodont, Paris). If an accident does occur, and blood or body fluids from one individual contaminate the mucous membranes or eyes, or the skin of an individual (usually a health care worker) is punctured by a contaminated 'sharp', then an immediate response is necessary. The first consideration is to deal with the site of contamination. If the eyes are involved they must be washed immediately with copious amounts of water or physiological saline, using an eye-wash kit. If skin has been punctured, encourage bleeding from the site of injury. Wash the site of injury thoroughly with soap and warm water, but without scrubbing, as this may further damage the contaminated area.

The incident must be reported to the senior clinician on the premises, who should:

- Take steps to identify (if possible) the source of contamination, if not already known.
- Decide if an accident record should be completed.
- Consider if attendance at the local casualty department is necessary. A decision can then be made, for example, on whether hepatitis B gamma globulin need be administered (this must be given within 48 hours of the injury).
- Consider seeking further advice from the local public health laboratory or District Medical/Dental Officer.

It is useful to complete a contamination report, so that the sequence of events and the action taken can be accurately recorded. This should list the information shown in Figure 7.3.

Post-operative bleeding

Persistent bleeding after an extraction or any other surgical procedure may result in patients contacting the surgery for advice several hours later, when their concern is rising. It is important to reassure them, and to inquire if they have been mouth-rinsing or applying pressure to the area by biting on a rolled cotton handkerchief. Calming them is an important first step, as anxiety raises blood pressure. In the vast majority of cases it is helpful to examine patients to put their minds at ease, as well as to clean their mouths of excessive clot, and if necessary to place sutures across the socket or surgical flap. The source of post-operative bleeding is often from soft tissues, particularly if the extraction has not been a clean one or the surgical flap is torn at the margins. It is often best to place an extra suture or two across a difficult extraction socket, or carefully to resuture a flap that has been difficult to reflect.

Name:

Date of Birth:

Position:

Date and time of injury:

Date and time reported:

Site of injury:

Bleeding from wound:

A + E department treatment provided:

Patient's name and address:

Signature of senior clinician:

Figure 7.3 The information to record at the time of injury. This information should be kept in a safe place such as a personnel file as it may be required at a later date.

In the case of a socket that does not stop bleeding after suturing a bleeding source from bone is likely. This may be controlled by the placement into the socket of some ribbon gauze soaked in saline, which is left for a few minutes. Alternatively, the placement into the socket of one of the haemostatic dressings, such as Surgicel (Johnson and Johnson Medical, Ascot, UK), which can be left in the socket may be helpful.

Finally, in cases where bleeding is profuse, making placement of Surgicel and its equivalents difficult, this may indicate that arterial bleeding is involved or that there is some other underlying pathology. In this instance, packing the socket with ribbon gauze soaked in Whitehead's varnish (which can be made up by a pharmacist) will often apply the pressure needed. If this arrests the haemorrhage it can be left for a few days, and the patient can be asked to return for the socket to be redressed less firmly with a standard socket dressing, such as BIPP on ribbon gauze, to allow healing to progress. In cases of excessive post-operative haemorrhage referral to the local consultant oral surgeon may be indicated, and the need for haematological investigations, such as a coagulation screen as well as a full blood count, should be considered.

Dry socket

The cause of dry sockets is still unknown; but it is obvious that some patients are more prone to them than others. Elderly patients who have a difficult extraction may suffer with a subsequent dry socket, particularly if little bleeding occurs immediately after the extraction. In addition, mandibular extractions seem to produce more of them than maxillary extractions. It is apparent that the more sclerotic and inflexible the bone is around a tooth, the chances of dry socket occurring after the extraction of that tooth increase.

A dry socket is different to an infected socket. A dry socket is due to a lack of bleeding into the socket, leaving alveolar bone of the socket wall exposed to the oral environment, which produces pain as soon as the local wears off. An infected socket initially forms a normal blood clot, which in a few days breaks down, and as a consequence becomes painful. The infection in the socket may be due to a foreign body, such as calculus, or a piece of fractured bone or tooth. The treatment is to remove the degenerating granulation tissue with a curette or excavator (under LA) and irrigate the socket thoroughly with sterile saline. For dry socket it is important to irrigate the socket thoroughly to remove all food debris, and then to dress the socket gently with BIPP on ribbon gauze that is also soaked with a few drops of chlorbutol to act as an obtundant. This is removed a few days later, and evidence of granulation tissue in the socket is sought.

There are proprietary products for dressing dry sockets readily available to dental practitioners, and these provide an alternative to ribbon gauze. In those sockets that are resistant to healing it may be necessary to explore surgically and induce bleeding from the bone walls by scraping an instrument along them, and finally to try to close the socket entrance slightly using a horizontal mattress suture, to protect the new blood clot and to allow healing.

In some patients it may be necessary to supplement the local measures with systemic antibiotics. Amoxycillin (250 mg three times a day for 5 days) and/or metronidazole (200 mg three times a day for 5 days) should be sufficient in the majority of cases.

Prescribing in dentistry

There are three ways to provide medication for patients who are undergoing dental treatment. The first is to recommend a drug that can be bought over the counter. This is cheaper for most dental patients than issuing a prescription, unless they are exempt from prescription charges. The second is to issue a private prescription to the patient, who pays the full cost of the drug plus a dispensing fee. This can be done for a prescription-only medicine that is not listed in the Dental Practitioners' Formulary (DPF). The third is to issue a National Health Service (NHS) prescription, which will be necessary if the drug can only be dispensed on the written authority of the dentist. Patients currently exempt from prescription charges under NHS regulations include the following:

- those under 16 years of age
- those under 19 years of age and in full-time education
- a man/woman who has passed the age of retirement
- someone who holds a current prepayment certificate
- someone who holds a current Family Practitioner's exemption certificate
- someone who is in receipt of Family Credit or Income Support, or holds a current exemption certificate
- someone who is a war/service pensioner holding an exemption certificate.

When prescribing in general dental practice the dentist, if treating the patient under NHS terms and conditions of service, will only be able to use the drugs listed in the Dental Practitioners' Formulary (DPF), which is found at the back of the British National Formulary (BNF). In hospital practice dental practitioners are not restricted to the drugs listed in the DPF, as it is recognized that clinical circumstances are often different and that to limit drug access would be inappropriate. The BNF lists all medicines currently available to patients on prescription or otherwise in the UK, and is a very useful reference in clinical practice. It is sent to all Doctors and Dentists free of charge, and is updated every six months.

Good prescribing practice

Drugs should be prescribed only when there is a definite indication, and in all cases the benefits of administering the drug should be balanced against the risks involved. In addition, the cost of different drugs that achieve the same therapeutic effect can vary widely, so it is advisable to bear cost in mind. To this end it is recommended that generic (non-proprietary) titles are used when writing a prescription. Proprietary titles are those followed by the symbol®, and are seen where the drug name is also a trade mark. Prescription-only medicines have the letters PoM placed before the drug name in the BNF. The prescription must be written in ink, be dated, show the patient's full name and address and be signed by the prescriber. The drug details should be written in English; but some still do use Latin abbreviations (for example qds for 4 × daily). When a clinician signs a prescription the legal responsibility for that action lies with that clinician, even if he is carrying out the request of another practitioner; therefore it is important to be sure that you are in possession of all the facts before signing. When prescriptions are to be signed by trainees the name of the principal who is responsible for the trainee must appear on the stamp at the bottom of the form. However, the prescribing clinician can print his or her name under the signature box, and so avoid confusion for the pharmacist.

A private prescription can be issued for drugs that are not listed in the dental practitioners' formulary, or for those undergoing private treatment; but this type of prescription can be expensive. Before issuing a private prescription it is advisable to telephone the local pharmacist and tell her or him that you would like to prescribe a certain drug. Ask them if they stock it, and what the charge for it, on a private prescription, would be. If the patient is willing to pay the charge (including the cost of the drug and the dispensing fee) then you can advise that the patient will be arriving shortly with the prescription. When issuing a private prescription it is important to follow the accepted method of prescription writing in English on practice notepaper. The dentist must sign it and stamp it with the practice stamp. However, it is worth noting that owing to increased NHS prescription charges it may be cheaper to issue a private prescription for the routine penicillins and metronidazole so often used in dental infections. A discussion with the local pharmacist may be helpful.

Adverse reactions to drugs

Rarely, a general dental practitioner may find that a patient develops a hypersensitivity reaction to a recommended or prescribed drug. When this occurs it is worthwhile reporting it to the Committee on Safety of Medicines (CSM). Yellow prepaid cards are issued in the back of the BNF which can be used for this purpose. It is also interesting for the dentist to request from the CSM a computer printout of the previously reported adverse reactions to this drug.

When a patient returns with an adverse drug reaction it is advisable to contact the medical practitioner (GP), to let him know and seek his advice. In all probability the GP will wish to see the patient; but he may advise you on steps that you could take. However, be sure any drugs recommended by the GP are listed in the DPF.

The most likely type of reaction that a dentist may see is a delayed hypersensitivity reaction, where the patient develops a skin rash a few days after starting a course of drug therapy. This responds in most cases to a course of promethazine hydrochloride tablets 10–20 mg three times daily after discontinuation of the original drug. However, the rash may be due to one of the exanthematous fevers developing coincidentally, and this is one of the reasons for informing the GP in such cases.

Prescriptions for the elderly

When prescribing or recommending drugs for the elderly it is helpful to remember that the ability of the older patient (over 65 years) to cope with drug therapy varies considerably. Elderly patients tend to take at least one drug for each ailment, and the number of drugs increases as they grow older. In addition, this section of society is exposed to gradual isolation as relatives and friends die, which places them under further stress for which they may seek additional drug therapy, including psychotropics. This may explain some of the behavioural changes seen in elderly patients. Moreover, the confusion often observed in the elderly may itself be an example of an adverse drug reaction, and may be caused by any of the commonly used drugs. It is also noteworthy that the presence of oral ulceration in the elderly confused patient may be due to retaining a tablet in the mouth, because swallowing is difficult for some elderly people.

The effect age has on drug metabolism is to reduce the rate of renal clearance, and this in turn can allow blood levels of a drug to build up in the body. In addition, bleeding associated with aspirin or other non-steroidal anti-inflammatory drugs tends to be more common in the elderly, and the outcome can be unpredictable. Therefore when prescribing for this section of the population it is useful to restrict your choice of drugs to those with a low incidence of side-effects. Also, it is important that instructions to the patient or carer are clear, and ideally the time of administering your drug should coincide with any concomitant therapy. Fortunately, the dentist will not be required to prescribe for the elderly very often; but when prescribing is necessary then it is useful to bear these points in mind.

Antibiotic prophylaxis

The prevention of infective endocarditis from dental sources has become much easier for the dental practitioner over the past decade, owing principally to the wide use of orally administered preparations. The dental procedures that require antibiotic prophylaxis against infective endocarditis include extractions, scaling, surgery involving the gingival tissues and endodontic procedures. When contemplating treatment involving antibiotic prophylaxis it is worthwhile also considering using a pre-treatment rinse of 0.2 per cent chlorhexidine gluconate mouthwash to lower the microbial population.

Regime 1 For patients who require dental treatment under local anaesthesia and are not penicillin-hypersensitive or have not received more than one course of penicillin in the past month, the following regime is recommended. This is suitable for those requiring antibiotic prophylaxis, including those with prosthetic heart valves who *have not* had endocarditis.

- Adult – 3 g amoxycillin orally 1 hour before procedure
- Child 5–10 years old – half adult dose orally
- Child under 5 years – quarter adult dose orally.

Regime 2 For penicillin-hypersensitive patients or those who have received a course of penicillin more than once within the past month oral clindamycin is recommended in the following dosages:

- Adult – 600 mg orally 1 hour before procedure
- Child of 5–10 years – half adult dose orally
- Child under 5 years – quarter adult dose orally.

Antibiotic prophylaxis in hospital

When general anaesthesia is required for dental patients who present no special risk there are two antibiotic regimes that can be considered. The first is administration of oral amoxycillin 3 g 4 hours prior to the procedure and again 3 g of oral amoxycillin as soon as possible after the procedure. For children 5–10 years the dose is halved, and for children under 5 years, quarter the adult dose. The other alternative, if the patient cannot wait, is to administer amoxycillin 1 g at induction **either** IM or IV, followed by oral amoxycillin 500 mg six hours later. Again the child dosages are halved in the 5–10 age group, and for the under-5s it is a quarter of the adult dose.

Special risk patients

Those patients who are deemed to be at special risk are those who require **general anaesthesia** and who **have had endocarditis or have a prosthetic heart valve**. These patients require 1 g of amoxycillin either IM or IV and 120 mg gentamycin IM or IV, followed by 500 mg amoxycillin 6 hours later.

When a patient is hypersensitive to penicillin or has received penicillin more than once in the previous month the antibiotic regime becomes complicated. In this case antibiotics can be given according to **one** of the following regimes:

1. Vancomycin 1 g given by slow IV (taking at least 100 minutes) followed by 120 mg of gentamycin IV at the time of, or 15 minutes before, induction. For a child under 10 years the dosage of vancomycin is 20 mg/kg and gentamycin 2 mg/kg.
2. Clindamycin 300 mg IV at least 15 minutes before induction or over 10 minutes at induction, followed by clindamycin 150 mg orally or IV 6 hours after the procedure. Child 5–10 years: half adult dose; under 5 years: quarter adult dose.
3. Teicoplanin 400 mg IV and gentamycin 120 mg IV at induction. For children under 14 years the dose of teicoplanin is 6 mg/kg and gentamycin 2 mg/kg.

The above drug regimes are recommended by the 1994 British National Formulary.

Orthopaedic prosthesis

The need for antibiotic cover for patients with prosthetic joints such as hips and knees is a more contentious area when considering cover prior to dental treatment. It has been stated by McGowan (1990) that there is no demonstrable need for antibiotic cover for these patients when they undergo dental treatment. Nevertheless, some orthopaedic surgeons still advocate cover to their patients. It may be useful therefore to follow locally accepted guidelines (if there are any) until the picture becomes clearer. A telephone call to one of the local consultant orthopaedic surgeons might be helpful. The current trend is not to provide this group of patients with antibiotic cover.

8

Medical emergencies

A. C. Crosby

Introduction

One of the most unpleasant aspects of emergencies in practice is that you always seem to be busy when they occur. Although serious medical emergencies rarely occur in dental practice, it is appropriate not only for the practitioner but also his or her staff to have a plan for dealing with a life-threatening event. This chapter outlines the commonest emergencies, and is meant to act as a framework around which you may assemble your own, possibly more complex, plans.

Resuscitation principles

Life support is now spoken of as basic and advanced. The latter form requires expensive machines and invasive techniques and, without regular rehearsal, using these becomes difficult. Basic life support is quickly learned, easy to rehearse and can be mastered by all the staff in your practice. It rests on the principles of keeping the patient's airway open, blowing oxygen into his or her lungs and, if the heart has stopped, pressing rhythmically on the sternum to depress two or three centimetres in an attempt to squeeze oxygenated blood around the body. This technique buys time, and can delay death by half an hour.

Basic cardio-pulmonary resuscitation (CPR) can be done by one person, but not for long – it is hard work. Changing position from chest compression to airway care is clumsy, and it is best to plan for at least two staff to take on this duty. Mouth-to-mouth breathing is possible, but possibly distasteful and potentially hazardous. A practice should have a basic resuscitation kit containing essential drugs (see Table 8.1), a selection of oral pharyngeal airways and a ventilation bag with a one-way valve (e.g. an 'Ambu bag'). A cylinder of oxygen is also required, and the qualified staff should have some experience in finding it and using it. Five minutes into

Table 8.1 Suggested essential drugs for medical emergencies in the dental practice

The following drugs are available as preloaded syringes, and should be kept in a clearly marked resuscitation box:

Atropine 1 mg in 10 ml (1/1000)
Lignocaine 100 mg in 10 ml
Adrenaline 1 mg in 10 ml (1/1000)
Adrenaline 1 mg in 100 ml (1/10 000)
Glucose 25 g in 50 ml
Hydrocortisone 100 mg in 2 ml.

The resuscitation box should also contain 500 ml of normal saline (2 bags) and 2 ampoules of diazepam 10 mg in 2 ml.

These drugs will help to stabilize an emergency situation prior to the patient's being transferred to hospital. Proprietary drug packs often contain more drugs than these, but some of those drugs should only be administered by personnel trained in their administration.

a serious emergency is not the best time to discover that no one can assemble the appropriate equipment.

Fainting

The commonest cause of a collapse in the clinical situation is fainting. The patient will become pale and momentarily unconscious. The pulse will not stop, but there may be limb twitching, which is self-limiting and should not be confused with epilepsy. A brief period of laying the patient flat is sufficient to allow recovery, after which there is no reason to postpone further procedures.

Cardiac arrest

Fortunately a cardiac arrest in the dental chair is infrequent, and is unlikely to occur without some warning, but it is probably most practitioners' recurrent nightmare. Although your training may have included practice with resuscitation dummies, a real human is different – wetter, floppier and much heavier, with ribs that crack if you press too hard. He or she will be unrousable to firm shaking, and although there may be respiratory efforts the carotid pulse will be absent. If you are near the airway, stay there and control it by sucking out saliva and pulling the jaw forward. Place an airway into the pharynx while calling for help. Minimize the drama and lessen the stress by encouraging those around you. Chest compression should occur about once a second, with one lung inflation to every five or six compressions. A dental chair makes a reasonable resuscitation couch, so resist the temptation to put the victim on the floor and ensure that the chair is adjusted to a height that allows chest compression to proceed efficiently. It is often very easy to put an IV cannula into the somewhat distended veins, and if you have enough help you should do this. Send for an ambulance, and do not give up even if the patient looks dead. Appearances can deceive, and although CPR cannot work miracles, you should share the responsibility with paramedics and the local hospital. Your job will be to ensure that the airway remains clear, the lungs inflated, and your assistants are pressing on the chest efficiently. Watch that their hand position does not wander away from the lower sternum, and look for the first signs of them tiring. Change assistants often. A cardiac arrest involves everyone in the vicinity, and possibly one or two volunteers from the waiting room as well. If nothing else, this will provide useful training for your staff – but ensure that you remain in overall charge.

Several problems may crop up. The airway of edentulous patients can be difficult to maintain without replacing their dentures. Vomit will be difficult to aspirate, and, although not invariably present during a cardiac arrest, may require manual removal if it consists largely of chunks of recently ingested food. In a hospital resuscitation room the ideal solution is to protect the airway with an endotracheal tube, but failing this a head-down position and continuous suction can often help. Clothing may also prove inconvenient, especially in the elderly who wear several layers. Do not waste time. Leave the clothes intact, as your chest compression will be equally good. Your assistants may grow disheartened by the lack of recovery; but console yourself with the thought that most victims of cardiac arrest die, and the only survivors are those who had someone helping them. Remember that basic CPR will not return a patient to consciousness. Remember also that small children will require less force when compressing the chest, but that compressions must be carried out at about 90–100 a minute. At the other end of the age scale the very elderly person can prove remarkably fragile. It is common in these cases to fracture several ribs during chest compression. The sternum may also fracture with an alarming crack. These injuries do not make CPR less effective; but neither do they improve patients' chances of survival.

Associated techniques

Defibrillation

Some practitioners may possess a defibrillator. The practice of using electric shocks in a clinical situation to depolarize a large mass of cardiac muscle dates back to 1962. Early models – long since superseded – used alternating current, but modern devices deliver a direct current shock from energy stored in capacitors. Recharging the capacitors takes place from the mains supply or integral nickel cadmium batteries. A solid state display screen shows the cardiac rhythm, which is detected through the defibrillator paddles.

The defibrillator is dangerous. It can deliver up to 400 joules, with currents of 35 amps flowing for a few milliseconds. The potential difference between the paddles may be of the order of 6000–8000 volts. All this is sufficient to spot-weld the paddles together, to kill yourself, or both.

The charge is delivered through the paddles, which are applied firmly to the skin over the patient's chest. Skin resistance is lowered by the application of conducting gel, or more commonly by the use of gel pads. When using a defibrillator it is essential to remember that these conducting pads do not touch – the current is meant to pass from pad to pad by way of the patient. Always ensure the patient is on a dry non-conducting surface, and warn those nearby to stand clear before discharge. The paddle handles are safe, and allow a one- or two-person operation; but no part of your body or clothing should be in contact with the patient. On discharge the patient's muscles will jerk, but this has never been shown to be a powerful enough effect to cause damage to teeth or dislocation of the TMJ.

It is highly advisable that you attend a course before purchasing a defibrillator. There are a number of arrhythmias that can respond to cardioversion, of which ventricular fibrillation is only one. Application of a DC shock at the wrong time or to the wrong rhythm is likely to make things much worse, by precipitating ventricular fibrillation or asystole.

Between the extremes of fainting and cardiac arrest are a number of conditions in which change in the heart rhythm causes a deterioration in the patient's condition. Spontaneous onset of supraventricular tachycardia is not uncommon. The patient may already be on medication, and will be well versed in her or his symptoms. The pulse will be very fast and regular, and the patient will feel breathless and somewhat unwell. Merely laying the patient absolutely flat may abort the attack; but if this fails, transfer to the local Emergency Department is appropriate. A similar prompt transferral will be required if a patient becomes drowsy and unwell with a very slow pulse. In such cases the problem is complete heart block, and the patient is usually elderly. Severe cases will require airway care, and may suffer asystolic cardiac arrest, so prepare for the worst while awaiting the ambulance.

Venepuncture

A common procedure in many such incidents is venepuncture. While a wise precaution, it is not always easy. You will not be giving large amounts of fluid quickly, so choose a small cannula (e.g. a pink Venflon 18 gauge cannula). This is more likely to get into a collapsed vein, and less likely merely to puncture the vein and cause a bruise. Old people in particular seem to have fragile veins, and, if you miss one, withdraw, press cotton wool over the puncture wound, and try elsewhere. Choose a big vein at the lateral antecubital fossa; but remember to prevent the patient bending the elbow afterwards, as this will kink and block the cannula. Some veins are difficult. Warming the arm and using an assistant to squeeze the upper arm instead of applying a tourniquet will help. Even when you are sure of getting into a vein, gently flick the target with the back of your fingernail, which will help the vein to distend. Your best chance is your first attempt, because further repeated venepunctures will cause anxiety in the patient and yourself, with a consequent deterioration in performance.

When your cannula is in place tape it in firmly; drying the surrounding skin with alcohol before applying tape is a helpful hint if the patient is clammy and sweaty. It is possible to put a cannula into a vein in almost any situation except in those patients with a lot of body fat. There are times when you cannot get venous access, and it is well to remember that in an emergency certain drugs can be given by alternative routes. In a cardiac arrest adrenaline and atropine can be given directly into the airway, but it is recommended that you use double the dose. In epileptic attacks diazepam may be given rectally.

Other causes of collapse

Acute asthmatic attack

Asthma is a common condition, and although sufferers will not come for dental treatment if they are very unwell, acute deterioration can occur with frightening speed. The patient will look unwell and will be fighting for air. The pulse will be rapid and the neck muscles will be working to assist the effort of breathing. The patient needs oxygen in large amounts given through a mask. Stay in attendance with the patient until an ambulance arrives, and do nothing to delay the patient's transfer to hospital. Asthma remains a significant cause of death. Patients may have inhalers with them, and one dose of their regular medication can do no harm. However, they should be gently dissuaded from over-use.

Diabetic coma

When patients have a history of diabetes, hypoglycaemia is the most likely cause of their becoming disorientated. Hyperglycaemia is a rare occurrence, and so in the emergency care of a diabetic who becomes confused and vague the first action is to administer some glucose orally (patients may carry sugar around with them in case they become 'hypo'), or intravenously if communication is difficult. The latter route will often allow the patients to recover composure very quickly – sometimes before the needle has been withdrawn from the vein. If this does not happen, the increased glucose loading will not significantly affect patients if they are hyperglycaemic, but a rapid referral to hospital is indicated.

Epilepsy

Neurological problems may present suddenly. Epileptic fits range from minor twitching of the limbs and transient disturbance of attention or consciousness to major convulsions in which consciousness is lost. Fits are self-limiting, and in the conscious case no action needs to be taken other than suspension of procedures. In the major convulsion, the problem is one of maintaining the airway. The patient's face will become alarmingly suffused and the breathing laboured and possibly obstructed. Turn the patient on his or her side, clear the mouth and nostrils by suction and if possible place an airway into the pharynx. If the teeth are clenched, do not struggle to part them – the fit will pass in a few minutes, and during this time oxygen by mask will help. The recovery follows, but the patient often feels confused and ill, and postponement of further procedures is sensible. A prolonged fit should be aborted by giving 5–10 mg of IV diazepam. Diazepam is also available in a form that can be given rectally; but in these unfamiliar circumstances the venous route will prove more reliable. An epileptic who has to be given diazepam should be transferred to the Emergency Department for a period of observation.

Transient ischaemic attacks

Elderly patients may suffer transient ischaemic attacks, small strokes in which some part of the body becomes numb and weak and the speech is slurred. There is no way in which recovery can be predicted in the first few minutes, and hospital referral is required. These attacks resolve in hours, although sometimes the blockage of the cerebral vessel progresses and becomes permanent. Consciousness is only lost in serious cases of brain ischaemia or haemorrhage, and maintaining the airway is the most important task. Brain haemorrhages may be accompanied by vomiting and fits, which are best managed in the emergency with basic airway care and IV diazepam.

Anaphylaxis

This is a rare, but potentially fatal condition. A variety of substances can precipitate it, ranging from antibiotics to lignocaine, and it occurs unpredictably, causing a rapid and progressive deterioration in the patient's condition. Antigens trigger anaphylaxis when they combine with IgE antibodies on mast cells, resulting in a release of histamine into the bloodstream and body tissues. The first symptom noticed by the patient is pronounced generalized itching, followed within seconds by the development of urticaria. A sensation of general distress envelops the patient, who is likely to have never experienced anaphylaxis. In some cases the condition may proceed no further, and following suitable treatment the patient may make an uneventful and swift recovery. However, in severe cases circulatory collapse, bronchospasm and pulmonary oedema may progress to cardiac arrest. It has been noted that individuals taking beta blocking drugs, for example for the treatment of hypertension, often prove difficult to manage.

The treatment of anaphylaxis lies in swift recognition of the symptoms. Remove what you feel may be the causative agent if it is possible to do so. Lay patients in a reclined position and give them oxygen. Administer 1:1000 adrenaline for adults and give 0.5 ml subcutaneously. Children require much smaller amounts: a dose of 0.1 mg per kg of 1:10 000 adrenaline should be used. Hydrocortisone and Piriton can be given intravenously, but their action is slower, and they should be considered a second line of treatment. Refer the patient to the local Emergency Department, and arrange ambulance transport. If time allows gain vascular access with an IV cannula and tape it firmly in place. Very low blood pressure will result in an unconscious patient with a feeble pulse, and in such cases 500 ml dextrose saline or normal saline should be given over a ten- to fifteen-minute period through the cannula. Even if one is not giving fluids, the cannula will be useful. Adrenaline wears off within minutes, and a second or third dose may be required if the patient again deteriorates.

Death

Despite all your preparation and efforts, the patient may die. After being certain that there are no heart sounds for one minute and that respiration has stopped, leave the body where it is if possible. Do not remove airways or IV cannulae, for the puncture wounds will leak. Your first duty is to preserve the dignity and privacy of any relatives present, who will almost certainly want to see the body, if only momentarily, before its removal is arranged by the police and the ambulance service.

Action immediately following a death

Thank your staff for their help. Find a private place and discuss briefly what happened. Rearrange your other patients to allow a period of deliberate relaxation. Do not continue as if nothing had happened. You should use this period to write up full notes of the incident, and if possible speak to the patient's general medical practitioner by telephone. You will also find it helpful to speak to the Coroner's Office and your Defence Society. If relatives were not present, prepare yourself for their arrival. Grief and emotional shock may show themselves as aggression and wild accusation. Keep a witness with you and avoid confrontation.

Subsequent actions

Expect to be called to Coroner's Court; if called, you cannot refuse. Take your original notes, and, if something went wrong, say so. Attempts at a cover-up are invariably unsuccessful. Coroners' Courts have been established for eight centuries in this country, and they now function as an excellent system for investigating death. A Coroner may be medically qualified, legally qualified, or both. It is his or her duty to ascertain the cause of a person's death, returning such verdicts as 'death by natural causes'. It is also possible for the Coroner to return a verdict of 'death due to lack of care or medical negligence'. Coroners have far-ranging powers, and if criminal activity is suspected they may refer a case to the Crown Prosecution Service. Being aware of these facts will enable you to approach attendance at an inquest with the gravity it merits. At an inquest you will give evidence under oath, and you will be expected to answer questions both from a Coroner and possibly from the relatives of the deceased or their legal representative. As with any court appearance, you must stay with the facts and be prepared to stand your ground. Do not hurry and do not bluster. After the inquest, anticipate the possible arrival of a solicitor's letter accusing you of negligence. Do not panic, for you will have solicitors on your side too. Respond promptly and remain courteous, and release your notes if they are requested.

Conclusion

Finally, keep abreast of developments and put time aside to train your staff at regular intervals. The unpredictability of serious emergencies can add spice to life, and if you deal with them competently the resulting increase in your self-confidence and the morale of your staff can be very gratifying.

9

The acute TMJ

P. S. Rothwell

Introduction

The temporomandibular joint (TMJ) causes few problems despite the complexity of its structure, the wide variations in its working environment and its susceptibility to the general diseases and disorders that can affect any joint. Yet, when TMJ problems do occur, they can offer some of the most demanding diagnostic challenges. Almost all TMJ and TMJ-related disorders have attracted controversies about their aetiologies and treatments at some time or other, and in-depth discussion of all theories and treatments will not be attempted in this chapter. Nevertheless, there are some acute problems associated with the TMJ with which a general dental practitioner will be confronted. The treatments described here are those required to give relief from the acute symptoms, and unless practitioners have engaged extensively in postgraduate educational courses devoted to TMJ problems they would be ill-advised to attempt treatments beyond the minimum necessary to make patients comfortable. Although the clinical techniques described in this chapter are simple, it is necessary to devote some space to the issues from which they derive their rationales.

It is important to appreciate that acute problems may arise in two basic conditions:

1. Where they arise *de novo* without any predisposing factors. Typical are problems arising as a result of direct or indirect trauma. In such cases, patients are usually able to correlate specific incidents with the onset of the symptoms and are able to confirm the important diagnostic point that the joint symptoms arose immediately following the incident.
2. Where they are acute exacerbations of an underlying chronic condition of which the sufferer may not have been aware. An example of this is acute pain from a TMJ which has condylar erosions, possibly resulting from years of chronic trauma. In

these cases, patients may neither be able to identify a specific exiting factor nor be aware that the joint had been partially destroyed or compromised for some time.

Basic anatomy

The anatomy of the TMJ is well described in many standard texts, but the classical description by Rees (1954) has stood the test of time. This short description outlines the main features relevant to acute problems. The TMJ has three special features when compared with other synovial joints. First, the TMJs are the only paired joints in the body where the movable elements, the condyles, are parts of a single bone, the mandible. In other paired joints the moving parts are on discrete bones. Thus, any irregularities or restrictions of movements in one TMJ will directly affect the movements of the contralateral condyle. Second, they are the only joints in the body the limitations of whose movements are determined not only by muscles, ligaments and the morphology of the articulating bones, but by another element, the teeth. Third, unlike the majority of synovial joints, whose articular surfaces are hyaline cartilage, those of the TMJ are fibrous cartilage.

The joint articulates the mandible with the temporal bone, and is divided into upper and lower compartments by a disc. The typical sagittal diagram of the TMJ gives the impression that a 'rod in a tube' situation exists. This is not so. The condyle is not a rod of uniform diameter, but a tapering bobbin shape. The condyles are angulated, so that the medial pole lies slightly distally to the lateral pole. The disc is traversed by two thickened bands (anterior and posterior) between which is an intermediate zone. In cross section the disc is not uniformly thick, but wedge-shaped, and thicker medially than laterally. Posteriorly, the disc is continuous with a bilaminar zone, which has an upper part consisting of elastic tissue attached to the posterior part of the glenoid fossa, and a lower part which is mostly collagenous and attached to the neck of the condyle. Laterally, the disc is attached to the joint capsule and to the lateral and medial poles of the condyle by discal ligaments. Anteriorly, it is connected medially to the superior body of the lateral pterygoid muscle and to the articular eminence and condyle, and laterally to the anterior slope of the articular eminence. The inferior head of the lateral pterygoid muscle is attached to the condyle. It has been shown by Juniper (1981) that the two bodies of the muscle act as antagonists. Rees (1954) described the overall shape of the disc as resembling a schoolboy's cap that enveloped the condyle, with a 'peak' anteriorly where it was inserted into the lateral pterygoid muscle.

It is important always to visualize the joint three-dimensionally to understand its functions and abnormalities. For example, the majority of disc displacements are antero-medial. This is not surprising because the wedge-shaped disc is thicker medially and would resist lateral, but would facilitate, medial displacements.

Functionally the disc divides the joint into two compartments. In the lower compartment the movements between condyle and disc are rotational, whereas in the upper compartment the movements are translational. It is the firm attachments of the disc to the poles of the condyles which make these rotational and translational movements possible. Supporting this idea is the fact that the common afflictions of the joint and disc are usually confined to the lower compartment.

In normal function the opening movement of the mandible (to about 16 mm inter-incisal distance) is basically one of rotation of the condyle in the lower compartment. As opening increases further the disc and condyle are brought forward by the lateral pterygoid muscle, a translation which is accompanied by forward movement of the disc along the floor of the fossa and along the slope of the eminence. This movement permits the mandible to trace the posterior margin of the sagittal envelope of movement.

When the mandible moves laterally, as when chewing, working-side (chewing side) and non-working-side conditions are described. In these movements the non-working-side condyle orbits around the working-side condyle, which, to allow this, needs to rotate around its vertical axis. However, the resulting movement is not one of pure rotation, and a small lateral component is introduced, which is referred to as the Bennett movement. The rotating condyle is located on the intermediate zone of the disc, and the wedge-shaped disc morphology possibly contributes to resist any medial movements.

Loading of the TMJ

The question of the loading of the TMJ has been the subject of much research. Barbenel (1974) postulated that potentially the site of occlusal load was critical. If located in the region of the molar teeth (and hence at the point of force application of the mandibular elevator muscles) there would be a minimal or no load on the TMJ, but, as the position of the occlusal load moved anteriorly, the load on the TMJ would increase by a lever effect. Further, the load on the TMJ would be determined by the position of the occlusal load in relation to the position of the occlusal plane in relation to the intercondylar axis. Although a simplistic overview, this is very useful when considering routine clinical treatments. It implies that one should strive for an occlusion where posterior bilateral chewing patterns are possible, and that the vertical dimension is maintained to ensure that the loading of the TMJ is kept, as far as practicable, within normal limits.

Examination and history

There are six stages to this aspect, namely taking the patient's history, observation of the patient, examination of the TMJ, examination of the muscles, examination of the mouth and examination of jaw dynamics. Because some are unique to TMJ diagnosis, the six stages will be discussed in more detail. It is useful to rehearse them until their use for every patient with a suspected disorder of the TMJ becomes automatic. A stethoscope is essential to interpret TMJ sounds adequately. A bell-end is preferable to one of a diaphragm type, because the latter can confuse sounds of hair movement with those of crepitus. A stereo-stethoscope has one bell attached to each earpiece, and is useful in identifying deflective or premature contacts (the bells are located over each maxilla, and patients are asked to tap their teeth together). It works on the principle that the clinician can locate the source of the sound by the difference in time taken for sounds to travel from a single source. Some clinicians suggest placing the bells over the TMJs, but, because there may be two sources of sounds (one from each joint), the stereophonic properties are lost, and the apparatus is being used as two standard stethoscopes.

The history

Sit at the same level as the patient to promote discussion; otherwise it is difficult to gain a patient's confidence and gain a true insight into the patient's problems and anxieties. The history is the key to the diagnosis. Of special interest are any occupational or recreational factors that affect the masticatory system either directly (such as singing or playing wind-instruments) or indirectly (such as weight-lifting). It is important to allow patients to describe their symptoms in their own words without being prompted by leading questions; only after this should the clinician start to ask such further questions as are needed to determine details such as the quality, intensity, distribution and existing factors relating to any pain. It is essential that the patient uses one finger only to outline the distribution of the pain, because the hand has the same surface area as the face, and if the patient indicates the distribution of the pain by using the outstretched palm and fingers the information will be of little value. The most common distribution pattern of pains related to TMJ disorders is radiation from the pre-auricular/TMJ area and into the mandible. Earache is commonly reported, and it is often difficult for a patient to distinguish pain from the ear or teeth. If there is any doubt, the general dental practitioner should have the patient's doctor check for any aural disorders.

Gradually, the history-taking should be directed to exploration of any personal situations which cause anxiety or worry. In general, patients in dental surgeries are not accustomed to being questioned about issues without apparent dental significance, and the subject must be approached with sensitivity.

Observation of patient

While taking the history, the clinician should note any relevant general signs. Evidence of nervousness or anxiety (chewed finger nails, nervous movements of the hands) or of musculoskeletal disorders (the patient's gait, flecking and ridging of the finger nails) are examples.

Examination of the TMJs

The TMJs are examined for tenderness by palpation both over the joints and via the external ears. Joint sounds should be auscultated during opening/closing and lateral movements, and identified as crepitus (crunching which occurs throughout all movements) or clicking; during vertical movements the latter should be classified, approximately, as early (within the first third of the opening movement), late (during the last third of opening movements) or multiple. If late clicks are detected they should be further explored by asking the patient to open and close the jaw after inserting the handle of a dental probe, or something of similar size, between the posterior teeth and noting whether the click can still be produced when the jaw movements are thus restricted. Experience indicates that late clicks which can still be elicited in such circumstances are extremely resistant to conservative measures. Assess asymmetries by viewing the patient's face from above (or from behind the chair with the patient recumbent), because the eye can detect differences in contours more easily when presented with an unfamiliar view.

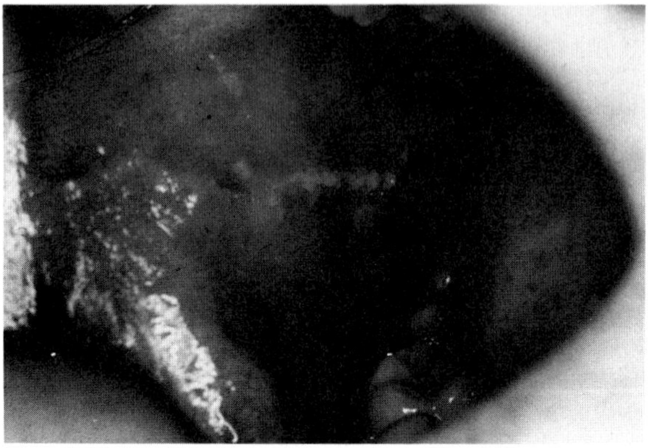

Figure 9.1

Examination of the muscles

Examine the masseter (palpate between the buccal mucosa and the outer cheek with finger and thumb), the temporalis (palpate with the patient clenching but trying to move the jaw laterally) and the lateral pterygoid. This last is difficult to palpate, and it is probably more meaningful if the clinician cups the patient's chin with the hand and asks him or her to try to move the mandible laterally against the resistance of the clinician's hand. Pain in the region of the joint when trying to move contralaterally is indicative of lateral pterygoid tenderness. It is important to test the integrity of both the facial and sensory nerves. Asking the patient to wink, wrinkle the forehead and smile will reveal any motor weakness, and normal sensory reactions should be tested by blunt probe, pinprick and stroking with teased cotton wool. This test should include areas innervated by each division of the trigeminal nerve and also those innervated by the first and second cervical nerves.

Examination of the mouth

The oral examination will include teeth, periodontal structures and mucosa. However, with suspected TMJ problems it is necessary to devote particular attention to signs of attrition of teeth and high spots on restorations – which suggest grinding habits, and to examining the cheek and tongue for evidence of mucosal ridges or scalloping – which suggest clenching habits (Figure 9.1). Observations of the tongue are best made when it is relaxed, because any ridges are masked by muscle contraction. Where indicated, comprehensive radiographic investigation should be carried out – by referral if necessary. As mentioned previously, it is important that patients with TMJ disorders should be able to chew bilaterally, and that there should be adequate posterior-tooth support. Although the concept of the 'functional' rather than the 'perfect' dentition is finding favour in terms of oral health and function (the 'shortened dental arch' concept), it is possible that the chewing patterns dictated by a shortened dental arch may lead to long-term degenerative changes in the TMJ due to overloading.

It is not appropriate to examine occlusal factors in detail at the stage when a patient presents with TMJ or muscular pains, because it is only when the painful episodes have resolved and the muscles and joints are relaxed that the true occlusal relationships can be determined.

Examination of jaw dynamics

Jaw dynamics vary greatly between individuals. In a routine examination the patient's opening and closing paths must be studied from both anterior and lateral aspects. Minor deviations from a straight vertical movement can be ignored, but marked differences of some 3 mm or more should be recorded. Probably the most common in patients with TMJ dysfunctions is protrusive deviation on opening. As was described earlier, the first opening movement of the mandible should be as a hinge, followed by translatory (protrusive) movements. In some patients this sequence is reversed, and translation occurs first, followed by rotation. When this is the case the patient's jaw should be gently opened and closed, guided by the clinician's hand on the patient's chin, within a range of approximately 15 mm inter-incisor opening, to demonstrate a normal initial rotational movement. Frequently, an early click will be alleviated by this. The patient is then instructed to practise this manoeuvre to restore normal patterns of opening. It is common for abnormal movements of the jaw to be perpetuated by patients who experiment to see if the click is still there. The maximum openings between the central incisors, both with and without pain and with and without sounds, should be measured, and, if one is using a Willis bite gauge in its reversed position, the thickness of the bite forks must be added. A simple estimation of whether there are restricted movements is that a normal jaw opening allows a minimum of three fingers to be inserted vertically (to half-way along the fingers) between the incisor teeth at maximum opening.

Radiography and other imaging

Radiography is not one of the more useful TMJ diagnostic aids unless gross lesions or deformities of the joint are present. The commonly-prescribed transcranial oblique view shows only the lateral pole of the condyle, and gives little information about either the condylar surface or the relationship of the condyle in the fossa. Further, this projection causes direct irradiation of the pituitary gland (Bishop, 1993) and the gross details which such projections reveal can often be detected just as well from a standard OPT film (remembering that this shows the medial pole of the condyle), so that this should be regarded as only a scout film. With dysfunction and degenerative changes, any radiographic changes detected are usually on the antero-superior part of the condyle (roughly between 5 and 50 degrees from the vertical plane) – the area of the condyle which experimental studies predict to be that most subject to loading (Barbenel, 1974). In TMJ dysfunction a flattening of the condylar contour can often be detected at that site, whereas with osteoarthrosis erosions or osteophytes may be noted. Specialized projections, such as the lateral transpharangeal, are not suited to general dental practice.

Other imaging methods, such as arthrography and magnetic resonance imaging (MRI), are restricted to hospital practice, but the information which these tests provide may very well be utilized by dental practitioners. Arthrography is cited as the most useful tool (deBurgh Norman and Bramley, 1990), and the author has known several instances where performing arthrography has by itself caused relief of symptoms. One of its great advantages is that the moving images can be seen in what could be called 'real time'. However, MRI may gradually replace arthrography in many circumstances, particularly where advanced splint therapy or restorative treatments are contemplated. MRI studies have shown that in normal populations (namely, those not complaining of any TMJ or TMJ-related problems), some 25–38 per cent show disc displacements (Kircof, 1987). Currently, imaging is expensive, but this must be weighed against the costs arising from faulty diagnosis. MRI is now of very high quality, and many diagnostic radiologists now restrict their interests to this medium. Figure 9.2 shows an MRI scan of a patient who attended with pain following prolonged use of an anterior repositioning splint, due in its turn to the patient's failing to return to the clinician who constructed it. The condyle is located just posterior to the eminence, and posterior movement is restricted by a mass of amorphous tissue which is becoming vascularized.

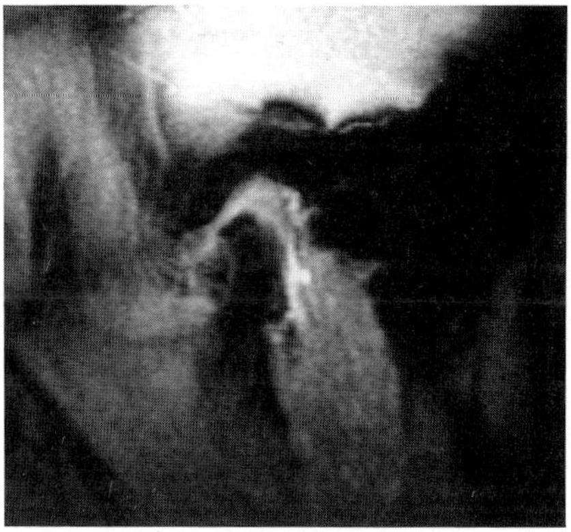

Figure 9.2

Classification of diseases

TMJ problems which require treatment may be divided into four types, viz acute trauma, dislocation, acute episodes of pain/dysfunction or osteoarthrosis, and acute presentation of systemic conditions. Each will be dealt with in turn.

Acute Trauma

Diagnosis

Acute trauma to the TMJ can be either extrinsic or intrinsic. In cases of acute extrinsic trauma the histories are of specifically-related events, either locally, for example fights, falls or injuries during ball games, or when TMJ trauma is part of a more general injury, for example a road traffic accident or some other major traumatic event. Either form of injury may produce a fracture, and when present it is impossible to palpate any joint movements. The joint is painful and tender and may be swollen, and the acute inflammation of the capsule restricts movement, so that when the patient opens the mouth the mandible deviates towards the affected side. The posterior occlusion is gagged. Where fractures are detected, treatment will be undertaken in hospital. Where no fractures are detected, the patient is advised to rest the jaw, prevent the joint from becoming cold (wear a scarf if out in cold winds) and eat a soft diet. External heat is helpful, and physiotherapy may be indicated.

The jaw movements of a patient whose TMJ has been traumatized should be monitored on a regular basis. An intra-articular haemarthrosis caused by the trauma may give rise to granulations in due course, with attendant restrictions in movements. Patients may not detect the gradual onset of such restrictions until they become quite severe.

Treatment

In cases of intrinsic trauma the patient can usually remember some specific event, such as yawning, stretching wide to bite into fruit, or getting the teeth stuck together by extremely sticky toffee, that has caused acute pain and a 'wrong bite'. In these cases there is dislocation of the disc, with a resulting temporary disturbance of the occlusion. In most instances, reassurance, advice and rest will result in resolution of symptoms. This may not be so rapid, however, in a patient who exhibits a marked parafunctional habit. Commonly, joints so traumatized develop clicks, the position of these in the movement path depending on the location of the disc at the time of injury. Such patients may require additional aids to recovery, such as a simple splint. The potential role of trauma in the development of dysfunctional symptoms will be discussed later.

Dislocation

Diagnosis

What is usually described by patients as a 'locked' jaw can be of two types: first, where the jaw is locked in an open position and cannot be closed (dislocation), and second, where the jaw is closed, or partially closed, and cannot be opened; the latter is a symptom of dysfunction, and will be discussed with that condition. With dislocation (which may be uni- or bilateral and either acute or chronic), the condyle has moved anterior to the eminence. There are various causes, including some that are post-traumatic or drug-related; but dislocation may be spontaneous. Usually, chronic dislocations are associated with tissue changes, such as a loose capsule or ligaments and condylar wear. Recurrent dislocations can be particularly troublesome in elderly persons living alone or in the mentally handicapped. Such patients can be referred for specialist opinion, with the possibility of surgical intervention.

Treatment

Instances of acute dislocation may be encountered in general dental practice during extraction of particularly resistant lower molar teeth, when extracting lower molar teeth in children under a general anaesthetic (although the latter procedures are becoming fewer with the improvement in oral health), or when taking impressions for the elderly. If such a dislocation is detected, reduction should be performed immediately, using the well-known manipulation of exerting downward and backward pressure in the lower molar region and elevating the anterior part of the mandible. If a patient presents with a dislocation only after it has been established, reduction will need to be undertaken under anaesthesia, and the opening will have to be restricted for a period subsequently. Thumbs should be protected during reduction attempts to prevent their being bitten by sudden reflex closing of the mandible after reduction.

Acute episodes of pain/dysfunction or arthrosis

Background

Dysfunctional and degenerative (arthrotic) problems are the two most common afflictions affecting the TMJ in the developed countries (this does not apply to Third World populations), and for their treatment it is necessary to have knowledge of the incidences of joint sounds and of parafunctional habits (bruxism) in general populations not complaining of any problems. Table 9.1 shows the results of examination of 500 patients attending a general dental practice for routine checks and who were not complaining of any TMJ or TMJ-related problems, and of a sequence of 500 patients attending a hospital clinic specializing in TMJ disorders (Rothwell, 1980).

From the incidence of joint sounds in 'normal' patients it is clear that many are unaware of and, therefore, unconcerned by the TMJ sounds detected by the clinician – a finding reported by many workers. However, the patients presenting in the TMJ clinic were aware of the majority of the sounds detected clinically. The presence of 'symptomless' TMJ joint sounds is a matter which should be appreciated at all times when diagnosing TMJ problems. The combination of sounds, pain and trismus is a classic triad which is often quoted in the literature. However, because of the somewhat capricious nature of the presence of sounds, and the sometimes nebulous connection between the sounds and the other symptoms,

Table 9.1 Incidence of TMJ sounds, bruxism and nature of onset of symptoms in study populations

	A. Incidence of TMJ sounds (%)			
	Normal subjects		*TMJ patients*	
	Aware	*Detected*	*Aware*	*Detected*
Male	9.2	25.3	71.1	79.4
Female	16.2	21.5	72.2	78.8
	B. Incidence of bruxism (%)			
	Normal subjects		*TMJ patients*	
	Aware	*Detected*	*Aware*	*Detected*
Male	12.7	26.3	43.3	72.2
Female	23.2	41.2	47.5	82.6
	C. Onset of symptoms (%)			
	Pain/dysfunction		*Osteoarthritis*	
	Males	*Females*	*Males*	*Females*
Acute	47.3	52.0	43.5	42.9
Chronic	39.2	34.9	52.2	44.4
Unknown	13.5	13.1	4.3	12.7

it is useful to consider the other symptoms on their own merits, and not to associate them with the sounds until a positive correlation can be established (Rothwell, 1987). It is interesting that the above figures for the incidences of joint sounds are comparable with incidences of disc displacement in normal subjects shown by MRI (Kircof, 1987).

The presentation of bruxism is quite different. Although many normal patients are unaware of bruxism, even though they exhibit clear clinical signs of parafunction, patients with TMJ problems are equally unaware of the habit.

Additionally, it can be observed that, although there is no sex-related difference in the incidences of clicking sounds, there is evidence of a significantly higher incidence of bruxism in females. This suggests that the higher incidence of females seeking treatment might in some way be influenced by their greater incidences of bruxism. The clinical significances of the undetected bruxist habit are considerable. Often, a patient will indicate that a specific traumatic event marked the start of problems – perhaps a minor event such as a yawn. Normally, the pains from such minor trauma resolve naturally within a day or so, owing to pain-enforced rest. In a bruxist, however, the situation can be perpetuated by the underlying hyperactivity of the masticatory muscles. Quite commonly this is seen when symptoms of dysfunction occur after a prolonged session of restorative dentistry or minor oral surgery.

In Table 9.1 the term 'detected' in relation to bruxism means that there were clear clinical signs of a bruxist habit. When a grinding habit is present, the pattern of tooth wear is usually quite distinctive, and the incisal edges and canine tips are ground down so that the patterns of wear on the upper and lower teeth match perfectly. It is important to remember, though, that teeth that have been worn by attrition reflect the end-product of historical events. Such tooth wear is irreversible, and its presence is no proof that the patient is indulging in a grinding habit at present. Consequently, it may be difficult to identify a direct relationship between bruxism and the presenting symptoms. Ridging of the buccal mucosa and tongue, however, are reversible conditions, and indicative of a current, on-going tooth-clenching habit.

The detection of a tooth-clenching habit in a patient who is unaware of it is complicated by the fact that it is a silent process, whereas cohabitants of tooth grinders can often hear the tooth-grinding (sometimes at a level which disturbs a cohabitant's sleep so badly that it leads to domestic strife). Although evidence of tooth grinding may not be elicited at a first consultation, it is common for patients to report at later visits that parents or siblings recall hearing them grinding in earlier years. In the author's opinion, it is prudent for dental practitioners to assume that every patient is a bruxist until proven otherwise. A 'false positive' from this approach will cause far fewer problems during routine dental treatment than will a 'false negative' from the alternative approach which **assumes** that a patient is not a bruxist.

There is overwhelming evidence that bruxism is a major factor in relation to problems in the TMJ–muscle complex. The two major forms of the habit – grinding and clenching – produce different outcomes. Grinding habits are associated more with clicking and remodelling of condyles than are clenching habits, which are more associated with degenerative lesions of the condyle and a resulting crepitus. Probably this is because of the intra-articular conditions which these habits create. During grinding the mandible is constantly translated backwards and forwards, with the disc occupying a position between the eminence and the condyle. During clenching, however, the disc and condyle are in their normal centric relation positions or have their positions dictated by the centric occlusion. Patients often state that the onset of clicking was acute; but, as was shown above, apparently symptom-free patients have clicking of which they are unaware.

There are two common non-joint-associated clinical situations created by bruxism to which clinicians should be alert. The first is where a patient complains of sensitivity to hot or cold or even of spontaneous periods of pain in a caries-free anterior tooth which is being traumatized by a tooth-grinding habit. The other is where molar teeth become sensitive to temperature changes or to percussion for no immediately obvious reason, where the sensitivity is in fact the result of a tooth-clenching habit which exercises its maximum effect on a slightly high restoration. Alertness to potential bruxism can save a great deal of diagnostic time in such circumstances.

To summarize, the important aspects of acute TMJ presentations in general dental practice are:

- Joint sounds may have been present before the acute episode, but are not necessarily noticed by the patient.
- Most patients attend because of the onset of symptoms other than sounds, namely pain and/or trismus.
- Merely asking patients about bruxist habits gives little meaningful information.

The importance of recording routinely the presence or absence of TMJ-related features, such as sounds or occasional locking, cannot be over-stressed. Sometimes patients complain that TMJ clicks that they have just noticed are direct consequences of some recent dental treatments, and unless their records show evidence that examinations of the TMJs were undertaken prior to the treatment, such allegations are virtually impossible to contest. Prolonged, time-consuming and extremely costly medico-legal actions have resulted from lack of such simple documentation in a patient's notes, as they have, also, from lack of documentation about parafunctional habits.

So far only dysfunction has been considered. The other common TMJ problem presenting in dental practice is osteoarthrosis (or arthritis). Osteoarthrosis is classified as being either primary or secondary, the latter usually secondary to trauma. Since the TMJ is not often affected, it is reasonable to consider the disease as secondary in nature. Most studies of TMJ osteoarthrosis, though, have not demonstrated significant histories of prior traumatic incidences. This leads to the possibility that most osteoarthrotic degenerative conditions of the TMJ are the result of chronic trauma, and, in the absence of evidence of specific traumatic events, the most likely causes of these are either a mutilated dentition or bruxism. Thus there is debate as to whether osteoarthrosis of the TMJ is a progression of dysfunction or whether it is a consequence of age and/or dentate status. In either case few patients complain about painless dysfunctions of

Table 9.2 Pain/dysfunction and osteoarthrosis: similarities in symptom patterns

Pain/dysfunction				*Osteoarthrosis*
Clicking	←	Chronic	→	Crepitus
↓		↓		↓
Pain ± Trismus	←	Acute	→	Pain
↓		↓		↓
Clicking	←	Chronic	→	Crepitus

their TMJs, and it is only when the TMJ becomes painful that patients present for treatment of dysfunction or osteoarthrosis.

An issue to be considered is what, in the cases of dysfunction or osteoarthosis, can be regarded a cure. Clinical experience demonstrates that when patients have been relieved of their major symptoms of dysfunction, usually pain and/or trismus, there are often residual TMJ sounds, but the incidence is that of a normal population. This suggests that most acute presentations of TMJ/muscle-related pains are temporary symptoms superimposed on underlying symptomless, chronic TMJ sounds. As a corollary, in osteoarthrosis, when the presenting symptom of pain has been relieved, the crepitus sounds remain. When treating the acute problems the general dental practitioner does not need, initially, to explore the underlying chronic troubles, but instead should concentrate on relieving the factors initiating the onset of pain and trismus.

Although the pathogenesis of the acute presentations of pain–dysfunction symptoms differ from those of osteoarthrosis, the clinical cycles exhibit similarities, viz symptom-free joint sounds (clicking in dysfunction and crepitus in osteoarthrosis) are overlaid with symptoms of pain and/or trismus. When the latter are resolved, the underlying sounds remain. Table 9.2 gives an overview of this concept. Although it is likely that the two conditions are age-determined states of the same condition, they will be dealt with separately.

Acute pain/dysfunction

Diagnosis

This condition has a variety of names, including pain/dysfunction syndrome, facial arthromyalgia, myofascial pain/dysfunction syndrome and craniomandibular dysfunction. It has a typical presentation of pain, trismus, clicking and locking in various combinations, and it is usually the association of these symptoms that leads to the diagnosis. Only a few years ago it was common to add to the diagnostic criteria the qualification 'in the absence of evidence of organic changes'. This absence usually meant that no radiographic abnormalities had been detected; the sophisticated imaging techniques available today have changed this claim, because they can demonstrate soft tissue changes undetectable on radiographs.

The most common symptoms presented in acute phases are the onset of pain, trismus, or locking or all three. This may then bring to the patient's attention the presence of clicking noises, or may exacerbate them. Probably the most common history is one where the patient has been aware of a clicking joint for some time, but suddenly, often in the morning on waking, becomes aware of a locked jaw, stiffness or pain. Because there are many conditions with pain and trismus as symptoms (such as the presence of a dental infection), it is essential that a comprehensive history and examination are taken to ensure that apparently typical dysfunctional symptoms are not arising from other sources. Remember that if any pain in the mouth is initiated or modified by hot or cold foods a tooth is involved somewhere, whatever additional problems may be present.

Locking, or 'sticking', as some patients describe it, occurs when the jaw is closed and cannot be opened. It is indicative of disc displacement. Patients often learn techniques to restore the disc's position by lateral manoeuvres, or even by 'knocking' the mandible on the affected side. From among the many potential causes of the dysfunction, many clinicians report a history of trauma to be important (Harkins and Martenay, 1985).

Occasionally, clicking itself can be the cause of a patient's seeking treatment, but this is unusual except when a loud (usually late) click has gradually become a source of embarrassment. Commonly, the onset of acute symptoms corresponds with a loss of the clicking. Similarly, a reduction of the acute symptoms is related to a return of the clicking. In most instances, though, there is a combination, where locking detected after awakening resolves and clicking returns.

Although the precise mechanism of TMJ clicking is uncertain, available evidence points to abnormalities of disc physiology/anatomy as being responsible. Where clicking is associated with occasional locking, it is reasonable to assume that there are circumstances (such as increased bruxist activity) that have temporarily induced locking. Overall, the relationships of disc, fossa and condyle are essentially normal. When spontaneous resolution is impossible, this suggests a situation where the disc is displaced to a degree that will demand treatment other than that to relieve acute symptoms. It is at this stage that advanced treatments are needed; but they are dealt with in more specialized texts.

Assuming that the diagnosis of the acute problem is established, it is most likely that the cause of the exacerbation of symptoms is muscle-related, and usually due to bruxism. The aim of initial treatment is to rest the affected tissues and relieve pain. First, the patient should be reassured that the problem is common, that it can be treated and that it is not sinister. This reassurance itself will help to reduce the patient's anxieties. Second, if any acquired movement paths have been detected, such as early protrusion during opening, the patient should be shown how to correct this and exercises should be prescribed to help (simple hand-out diagrams or photographs are very useful). Third, if there are any contributory occupational or recreational factors, these should be addressed. Usually, it is easy for a patient to give up temporarily or to reduce recreational activities, such as choir singing, but occupational factors are more difficult to reorganize or avoid. However, this is a disorder causing pain and discomfort, and if patients need rest from an occupational aggravation they should be treated just as with any ailments elsewhere in the body. Fourth, it is useful to ascertain what the patient eats or drinks before going to bed. It is not unusual to discover that patients drink stimulants, such as coffee, last thing at night. A change to a hot milk drink can be helpful in many instances. Fifth, if unilateral or anterior-tooth chewing patterns are present these should be corrected. Occasionally, these patterns will have developed because of lack of occlusion and/or sensitivity of certain teeth, and these should be treated by prosthetic or restorative means as a first priority.

Treatment

The initial treatment preferred by the author is the use of simple so-called occlusal splints. Whatever effect such appliances have in TMJ therapy, it is not by any splinting action in the traditional medical sense. Other descriptions, such as bite-raising appliances, imply that their effects are mediated via the occlusion, which is not necessarily the case. In fact, it is very difficult to define how such devices do produce their effects, because their presence stimulates the sensory nerves, directly or indirectly, of all tissues of the oral cavity, including the masticatory muscles, tendons and receptors of the TMJ and capsule. Further, all will alter the condyle–fossa relationship. Many designs of splint have been developed over the years. Some have occluded only the posterior teeth; others have been fitted with occlusal pivots in the molar region; others have

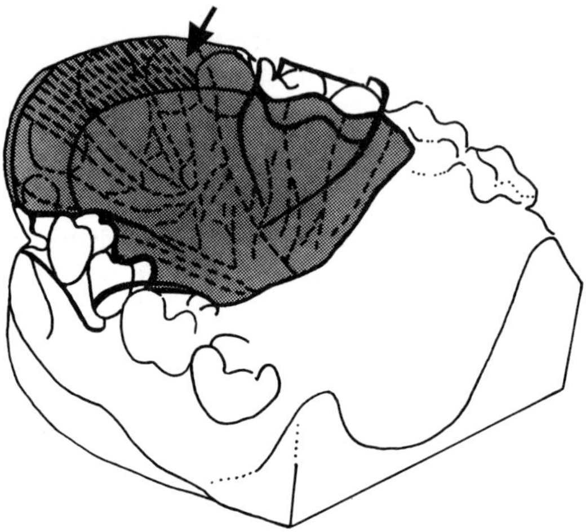

Figure 9.3 A simple anterior biteplane splint with an incisal bite platform but no ocdusal or incisal cover

names which indicate their functions, such as anterior repositioning and centric relation; and some carry the names of their designers. It is because of these various names that the author prefers to call those described for use here, 'simple' – they are, in comparison with other designs.

When clear evidence of wear on the incisor/canine teeth is seen, a grinding habit can be diagnosed. A simple anterior bite plane splint with an incisal bite platform but without any occlusal or incisal cover will be effective (although in some instances it may be necessary to extend the bite plane over the incisal edges because of occlusal relationship). Figure 9.3 shows the design. The bite plane is flat, and because of the classical pattern of tooth wear seen in tooth grinders, the lower anterior teeth usually occlude on the plane, with little or no grinding-in being needed. Retention is by cribs on appropriate teeth. Since the posterior teeth are discluded when the splint is in use, the cribs do not interfere with the occlusion. If there is no evidence of a grinding habit, but the mucosa of the tongue and/or cheeks shows ridges, the use of a soft resilient-material splint on the lower teeth will ease the problem in the initial stages. Both types of splint should be worn only at night. However, many stressed patients have daytime clenching habits. Common occasions are when driving in adverse conditions on motorways or when 'catching-up' to keep an appointment, and during periods of intense concentration at the desk or computer. When alerted to the situation, such patients can benefit from the occasional use of the soft splint at such identified times. Treatment will provide relief for approximately 90 per cent of patients. If it does not, it is wise to refer the patient for specialist opinion.

Although antidepressant drugs can be effective, many patients are averse to taking them unless they are absolutely essential, and the unsuspected dependence which developed from the use of minor anxiolytics a few years ago reinforces these fears. The drugs recommended (usually tricyclic antidepressants) are apparently safe, but have the disadvantage, when treating acute problems, that they need to be taken for some time before their effects are manifest. Their routine use for treatment of TMJ disorders is difficult to justify.

Rationale for simple splint treatment

The reasons for proposing the use of the simple splints preferred here are:

- They work well and quickly to relieve symptoms in almost 90 per cent of cases within 2–10 days.
- They have no irreversible effects if used as prescribed.
- Their fabrication is inexpensive and does not call for specialist technicians.
- They may be used intermittently over many years.

Bruxism is not a habit that exhibits a constant pattern of activity but one that varies with personal circumstances, and painful symptoms may regress spontaneously without treatment, either because the existing factors disappear, or because of self-limitation of jaw activity imposed by the patient as a result of the pain, or because reassurance has caused a reduction in the muscle hyperactivity. It is possible that simple splints merely accelerate the process, just as a bandage helps to rest a sprained ankle; and if they make the patient comfortable more quickly then their use is justified.

Aetiology

In many patients with TMJ dysfunction pain and trismus, Bessette and co-workers (1973) observed a doubling in length of the silent period (an electromyographic phenomenon). Similarly, Cox and co-workers (1982) showed, that in normal subjects, experimental bruxism can produce the same symptoms and similarly increase the silent periods. The time of the silent period reduces to within normal limits when pain and trismus are reduced in both patients and experimental subjects. Cox and Rothwell (1983) showed that when subjects performing experimental bruxism wear a simple anterior bite guard they do not develop pain or trismus, nor are their silent periods increased.

The upper and lower bodies of the lateral pterygoid muscle have different actions (Juniper, 1981), the upper part being active in jaw closing and the lower part in opening and protrusive movements, the two parts acting as antagonists. In an electromyographic study of the lateral pterygoid muscle, Juniper (1984) showed that in patients with painful dysfunction this reciprocal movement was replaced by totally 'bizarre' patterns, but in patients suffering only from joint clicking the two parts of the muscle exhibited the pattern noted in normal subjects. This suggests that the change from 'asymptomatic clicking' to painful dysfunction also involves muscular effects. Currently, there is more evidence that the causes of acute dysfunctional TMJ symptoms are muscle-based than that they arise from occlusal factors.

Prophylaxis

Dental treatments for patients with TMJ-related disorders should be undertaken with caution, because extended periods of mouth opening are well known to trigger periods of pain and limitation of movement. A rubber prop, or other device, used during treatment will help patients rest the teeth on the prop rather than maintain positive muscle activity to keep the mouth open, and thereby possibly precipitating post-operative discomfort and pain.

Psychological/psychiatric factors

Many of the muscle-related factors in patients with acute problems can be identified with the emotional upsets which are part and parcel of everyday living. However, consideration should be given to situations where the symptoms reflect a more deep-seated psychological state. Many years ago it was established that facial pain could be a manifestation of depression (Lascelles, 1966), and subsequent studies have supported this (Fine, 1971). It has been demonstrated that many patients who suffer from 'TMJ dysfunction' suffer also from disorders such as irritable bowel syndrome, migraine, dysmenorrhea and hay fever and other allergies (Berry, 1969). These aspects of TMJ problems have been studied in depth in recent years, and concepts of emotional influences have gained considerable support (Feinmann and Harris, 1984). It is not proposed to go further into this debate here, other than to state that such a consideration should always be in the dental practitioner's mind. If an underlying psychological problem is suspected, then referral is recommended, either to a dental consultant or to the patient's medical practitioner. The dentist's role is that of detecting any dental cause in what might be a non-dental disease. Other health care workers will depend on this vital part of the diagnostic sieve, and the opinion of the dentist is crucial. Before reaching decisions that a symptom is dysfunctional, emotional or of other non-dental origin, the dental practitioner should ensure that no stone is left unturned in the search for a possible dental cause. Comprehensive radiographic examination of relevant sites, vitality tests and exploration for cracked cusps are mandatory. Any patient with a suspected maxillary sinus involvement should be referred for a consultant opinion. It is with good reason that TMJ Clinics are often called diagnostic dustbins.

Most dental practitioners are uncomfortable when presented with symptoms that may be psychologically based or have a chronic nature, because they are accustomed to providing an immediate cure. A classic case is the construction of numerous complete dentures for a patient by successive dentists, each convinced of his own ability to succeed with a case which is basically one of patient intolerance. Some patients who present with TMJ and TMJ-related dysfunctions may well fall into a similar group whose primary problems are not dental, and the practitioner should be wary of undertaking a series of operative procedures in a relentless quest for a cure. The following guides for identifying a possible psychological background to orofacial problems might be useful, and are based on the author's own experiences.

There are grounds for suspecting underlying psychological factors in the following circumstances:

- Where pains are bilateral, always starting at exactly the same time and for no apparent reason.
- When patients use words that are not typical of those used to describe orofacial pains. The description of a dental pain as 'vice-like' is an example.

- Where the patient's primary complaint is that the 'bite feels wrong', although a preliminary examination shows a reasonable occlusion.
- Where there is insistence that a perfectly normal tooth, or even a sound area of alveolus, is the source of the pain.

Psychological problems associated with orofacial pain are fully covered in the literature (Feinmann and Harris, 1984; Lamey and Lewis, 1989).

Acute episodes of osteoarthrosis

Diagnosis

The International Classification of Diseases recognizes osteoarthrosis as a degenerative condition, whereas with an acute inflammatory involvement the condition is termed osteoarthritis. In the TMJ the degeneration is probably caused by chronic trauma due to overloading. The principal symptom is crepitus from within the joint, although, as was mentioned previously, the patient may be unaware of this. There is evidence that over a period of time the condition may resolve by remodelling of the condyle (Toller, 1973), perhaps because changes in the occlusion or the patient's habits reduce the load across the joint. When the condition undergoes an acute episode it is likely to be due to an inflammatory response, and these seem to be random and not related to the degree of destruction of the condyle. Great pain may be experienced by patients with minimal erosions, whereas extensive erosions may be pain-free for long periods. The cause of the pain is possibly irritation caused by osteophytes.

Treatment

Immediate treatment is to advise the patient to rest the joint by adopting a soft diet; local heat and, if necessary, either analgesics or non-steroidal anti-inflammatory drugs (NSAIDs) may be helpful. The use of a full-cover occlusally-balanced splint will effect rest by reducing the load, and, if necessary, such splints can be constructed to fit over full lower dentures. Long-term treatment will be to try to reduce the load by alleviating the effects of any bruxist habit or by restoring the occlusion if it is deficient. Fortunately, the response to these treatments is very good.

It is unwise to remake complete dentures when patients present with osteoarthritic pain until a comfortable vertical dimension has been established by means of adjustable splints. In many cases, where patients present with grossly worn dentures and an apparently gross deviation from what is considered a 'normal' freeway space, it is tempting to remake the dentures to restore normal criteria. However, this should be resisted until a pain-free vertical dimension has been established, lest the problems presented by the joint are compounded by difficulties commonly encountered by patients adapting to new dentures.

Acute presentation of systemic problems (arthritides)

Diagnosis and treatment

It is uncommon for the TMJs to be the most painful of the joints affected in systemic arthritides, even though there is evidence that they are affected in about 50 per cent of sufferers from rheumatoid arthritis (Ogus, 1975). Problems are sometimes encountered, however, usually during periods of exacerbation of the disease, and it is important that joints damaged by inflammatory disorders are not subjected to further trauma from overloading. Where the TMJs are not seriously affected, or where patients are known to be suffering from an arthritic disease, even in the absence of any TMJ-related complaints, it is useful to monitor the incisal opening routinely to detect any reductions that the patient may not have detected and to monitor the occlusion to preclude situations that would lead to overloading. Conservative treatment is the same as that in osteoarthrosis. If there is reduction of opening, the patient should be asked to undertake regular exercises to maintain the gape. Dental technicians are particularly adept at making acrylic trismus 'screws', which are very helpful to patients in such circumstances. However, where the TMJ exhibits evidence of more severe involvement, and advanced destruction is evident, there can be a loss of condylar support and, therefore, vertical height; this is accompanied by occlusal changes that result in the creation of an anterior open bite. In these circumstances, treatment by GDPs should be in collaboration with the appropriate consultants.

Conclusion

This short chapter has attempted to provide a simple guide to general dental practitioners confronted with acute problems of the TMJ. The treatments proposed have sound rationales which have been well tested over many years and shown to be effective initial treatments for use by practitioners without specialized training in the complexities surrounding the TMJ.

Basic rules that general dental practitioners should follow in the treatment of acute TMJ or TMJ-related problems are:

1. Decide on specific treatment protocols with well-documented rationales, and abide by them until such time as more effective and scientifically evaluated alternatives are demonstrated.
2. Decide an end-point (either in time or in treatment options) after which the patient will be referred if treatment has not been effective; do not embark on a succession of further treatments.
3. Ensure that any treatment fulfils the requirements for informed consent (Bullen, 1993), which are:

   - Patients must understand what the procedure involves, what it is intended to do, and the alternatives.
   - Patients must know what might happen if the treatment is not undertaken (i.e. that the condition might resolve spontaneously or that it might need alternative treatment).
   - Patients must be informed of all potential risks.
   - Patients must be informed of the chances of success.

   See Table 9.3 for an application of these requirements to simple splint treatment for acute TMJ pain.

Table 9.3 Requirements for informed consent as they relate to the nature of simple splint treatment for acute TMJ pain

Requirements for informed consent	*Application to simple splint therapy for acute TMJ pain*
Patient must understand what the procedure involves, what it is intended to do and what the alternatives are.	Construction of a simple removable device which is placed on the teeth to allow temporary rest of muscle and joint tissues. Most common alternatives are drugs, rest, more complex splints, physiotherapy.
Patient must know what might happen if the treatment is not undertaken.	Symptoms may improve spontaneously with time or may need alternative treatment. The splint probably speeds up relief of symptoms.
Patient must be informed of all potential risks associated with the treatment.	None reported that are not reversible if instructions (e.g. night use only) are followed.
Patient must know the chances of success.	Up to 90% chance of being effective, but will not prejudice further treatments if not effective.

Domiciliary care and special needs

Nigel Thomas

Introduction

In general, people have special needs only if they cannot receive care in the usual way. A blind person who can sit relaxed in the dental chair and receive conventional dental care is no more a case of special need than a sighted person. However, many people do have special needs when dentistry is involved, and for some, such as housebound patients, this means that care must be brought to them. Fortunately a dental chair is no longer necessary when providing such care outside the surgery, and apart from the X-ray unit, nearly all dental equipment is now easily portable, and transport is no longer the problem it was. Some problems of domiciliary care still remain, and these will be addressed in this chapter and have appropriate solutions provided for them. Treatment modes applicable to the surgery will also be described.

Personnel requirements

Although it is tempting to undertake domiciliary treatment alone on one's way home from the surgery, the presence of a Dental Assistant is essential. The assistant can support the patient's head, hold a torch, help with the improvisation of surgery routine (which differs in each situation) and still provide the usual clinical support. In addition, the presence of a relative or friend of the patient can be helpful in clarifying the medical history or explaining treatment or procedures. Moreover, someone who knows the patient well may be able to interpret his or her speech and wishes far better than the dental team, and, while probably not keen to stay during treatment, may be an invaluable communication link.

Appointments

The first visit can be crucial. The patient should have been contacted earlier to agree the time and date of the visit. Disabled people often have great patience, but become a little anxious if you are late. Many home visits bring an element of social contact as well, and the visit will almost certainly be a major event in the week. If patients are on the telephone, a short call before leaving the surgery will reassure them. Patients without a telephone need to be contacted by post in good time, and with them every effort must be made to be punctual.

The first visit should be an introductory one for both parties. The patient needs to meet you and your assistant and discuss treatment needs and costs. You need to take a history, make an examination and treatment plan, decide how you will carry out the treatment, and note lighting, patient position and the site of electrical points. When the visit is over, leave an appointment card, with the surgery telephone number and the next visit clearly marked. Bear in mind laboratory processing times when arranging the next visit, and check that it does not clash with the patient's hospital/clinic or District Nurse sessions.

Gaining access

Many elderly and housebound people live alone, with calls from relatives, Meals-on-Wheels and the Home-help services, in addition to any regular health visits. Fear of crime is usually great, and to make access easier it will first be necessary to gain the patient's trust. By showing that you are reliable, you can usually arrange for a back-door to be left open for your entry. A loud knock and an announcement of who you are will usually set the patient's mind at ease.

At the first visit it is helpful to have a friend of the patient present. Afterwards, arrangements can be made for access, often timing it to coincide with some other event. But do not arrange to come at the same time as the Meals-on-Wheels service, or else the food will be cold by the time treatment is complete.

Medico-legal requirements

Consent

Consent to treatment is the same for the housebound as for all other dental patients. Informed consent is required, and the patient must understand what form of treatment is to be provided. Another person, be they carer, relative or manager of a home, cannot give consent for adult patients on their behalf; but obviously they must be consulted and agree with the proposed treatment. At times it is necessary to provide pain-relief and other essential health care for a person who is unable to understand the procedures (for example someone with profound learning difficulties, or a patient who has suffered a major stroke). In such circumstances the proposed treatment may have to be agreed with another dentist or with the patient's doctor, so that two clinicians are in agreement over the proposed treatment; this may be important to satisfy medico-legal considerations that may arise if the treatment is questioned at a later date (Department of Health, NHS Management Executive Health Circular (90) 22: *Patient consent to examination or treatment*). Contact with the doctor should have already been made if there are medical complications. As with all aspects of dentistry, careful notes of all procedures are essential.

Chaperon

As mentioned already, a dental assistant provides much needed clinical support, but is also essential as a chaperon. On home visits one is on the patient's territory and surrounded by the patient's possessions. Elderly patients can become confused, and can mislay objects. The continuous presence of a third party may therefore prevent an accusation or even an unvoiced suspicion on the part of the patient that the dentist is responsible for the loss or breakage of some cherished article – which would immediately destroy the relationship being established. Any articles accidentally damaged by the dentist on home visits must be replaced, and it is worth checking the practice insurance to ensure that you are covered for home visits.

An uncooperative patient

A patient who becomes uncooperative during treatment can cause problems. Patients with dementia can have intermittent spells of confusion. If in doubt, postpone further treatment until co-operation becomes possible. Do not be persuaded by relatives to press on with treatment in the face of resistance by the patient. If dentures remain uncompleted, little is lost, as few confused patients are able to wear them. If tooth restoration is involved, then a referral to the

Community Dental Service or the Hospital Service for completion of treatment under sedation or general anaesthesia may be the only solution.

Choice of room

There is a common misconception that to achieve adequate cross-infection control the dentist must emulate the conditions in his practice. It is not necessary to treat the patient on a hard chair in the kitchen, where all surfaces can be swabbed down. Only the dentist and associated equipment will be in contact with subsequent patients, not the chair or the work surface. It is best to settle patients comfortably in their usual chairs in the living room, provided they have adequate neck and head support, and allow sufficient access for treatment. This is usually true of most domiciliary care.

On the other hand, it is ideal to use a firm, clean work surface in the kitchen for the preparation of materials – particularly impression materials, such as alginate, that require vigorous mixing, and then carry the loaded tray to the patient. Take advantage of auto-mixing impression materials (provided in gun form), and the ready-mixed light-cured restorative materials. Covering the work surface with a large paper towel greatly speeds the clearing-up time.

Obviously, it is unproductive to have the spirit-burner or hot-air Bunsen so far from the patient that wax has hardened by the time it reaches them. A convenient table near to the patient's chair is the best site. A small rubber mat, such as is sold for the floors of cars, provides a good non-slip surface and is also an effective insulator. Small gas-powered wax knives are now available that run off gas-lighter fuel and eliminate the need for a conventional burner. Somewhere is still required to support instruments, occlusal blocks and models, as well as spare wax, which may be hot. Water is usually needed, and the kitchen therefore remains the most convenient preparation area.

Posture and support

Success in domiciliary care usually depends on good access and patient posture. It is recommended that cushions are placed behind the patient's back, as far up as the base of the neck. This allows the head to fall back at an optimal angle. Occasionally the dental assistant may need to provide extra support by placing his or her hands behind the patient's head. Upper impressions should be taken

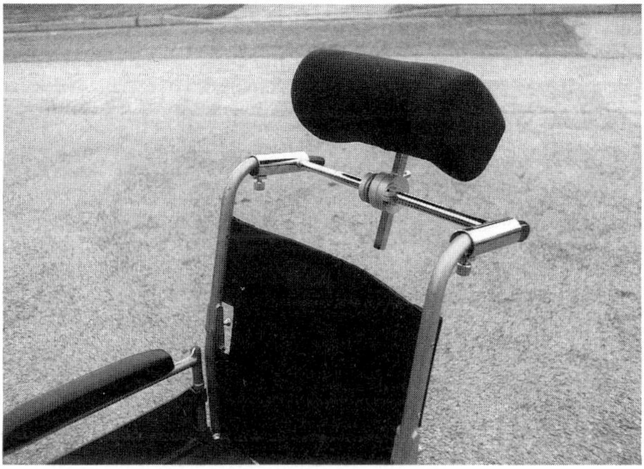

Figure 10.1. A vehicle-type headrest adapted to fit a dental chair.

from behind as usual, and the position of the chair and surrounding furniture should make this possible. Do not hesitate to ask to arrange the furniture as required – this is always accepted by the patient, who is normally delighted that treatment can be carried out at home. Lower impressions and the registration stage are best undertaken kneeling in front of the patient. A kneeling pad from a garden centre provides comfort for the knees, and the angle of working ensures a straight back and a relaxed posture.

According to the form of treatment, the position of the patient in the chair or bed is very significant. Prosthetics can be carried out with the patient in a variety of postures, but other types of restorative work require the patient's position to be varied according to the dentist's working practice. Conservation can be carried out from in front of the patient, but it can usually be completed more easily and to a higher standard the nearer the working position is to that existing in the surgery. A high-backed chair can give good support to the head and neck if a small cushion or rolled-up towel is placed at the back of the neck and the head is allowed to lean back. A wheelchair can be an excellent temporary dental chair if a headrest is attached to the handles (Figure 10.1) and placed in such a way as to allow the patient's head to angle back safely.

Problems with patients who are bed-bound can be overcome with a folding backrest. The patient can then be propped up in bed lying back against pillows on the backrest, and treatment can be provided from in front. A better solution is to use a light wooden board, approximately 10 inches by 4 feet 6 inches (250 × 1500 mm). The patient lies the wrong way round in bed, with the head projecting over the foot of the bed. The board is slipped underneath the patient, with a pillow or cushion on it to support the head. The patient's weight is sufficient to keep the board in the correct place. If the bed has a footboard or similar impediment, the patient is placed diagnoally across the bed with the head projecting out at the side.

Equipment

Light

Whatever the treatment, the first essential is light. Most people's homes, even in the kitchen, do not have lighting levels suitable for clinical dentistry. For occasional domiciliary work, a portable headlight of the type sold for caving is ideal, as long as the beam can be concentrated on the mouth. Generally, the greater the cost the more useful the light. A light with an adjustable beam width is ideal. Anglepoise lights are a possibility, particularly if the patient already has one available; but they are cumbersome to carry, and do not have a covered bulb for safety. A Daray 4000 light with a clamp on the end is the ideal solution. It is light and portable and provides a controlled illumination similar to a surgery light. The cost (in the region of £250) may be the major inhibition to purchase. If held by the assistant, a simple pen torch can be used for short visits, and one should always be carried in the domiciliary box, along with spare batteries.

The only place where extra light is unnecessary is in the hospital ward. Virtually all hospital beds have an adjustable reading light above the patient's head.

Power

Electrical power is essential for almost all dental procedures. Suitable extension leads, preferably of the type sold for computer or hi-fi use, with a single lead and plug connected to a block of three or four sockets, should be carried. Block multiple connectors holding two or three plugs together in one socket are not recommended. They can easily overload, as there is no fuse between them and the socket. The 3-pin 13 amp electrical socket is universal in the UK, but occasionally obsolete 5 amp and 15 amp round pin sockets are discovered in older houses. If necessary, a simple adaptor with a 5 or 15 amp plug on one end of a foot of flex and a 13 amp socket on the other solves the problem. Spare fuses and a suitable screwdriver should always be carried.

The first visit to the patient, for examination and treatment plan, must also be used for assessing the powerpoints in the chosen treatment room. Try to keep the distance between the socket and the equipment to a minimum, to avoid tripping. However, if power extensions of the type wound on a drum are used, remember to unwind them completely, to prevent unwanted heating from the still wound portion.

Hand instruments

A box is preferred to carry the required hand instruments and sundries. It should be light, capacious and capable of being sat on. The Mothercare Baby-box is a good choice. It is capacious enough to carry all necessary items. Soft airline-type travel bags are very useful for individual items of kit, such as light-cure guns, a selection of restorative resins, or an amalgamator or suction apparatus. If the bag has a shoulder-strap, its versatility is greatly increased.

To prevent the possibility of forgetting instruments, it is advisable to have standard set-ups, with a printed checklist card. If this is supplemented with an instrument tray for each patient containing essentials, such as mirror, probe, tweezers, cotton rolls and napkins, all covered with an aluminium lid, several patients can be seen on the same journey. Each clinician will choose a selection of instruments appropriate to his or her own mode of working, but there are one or two extra items which have stood the test of time despite their appearing unnecessary for home visits. These include a wide-bladed wallpaper scraper for smoothing and levelling registration blocks, a hobbyist's or engraver's mini-drill for trimming acrylic and for adjusting dentures, and a Camping-Gaz single burner with a spare cartridge. Acrylic trimming *can* be done with a cordless electric drill; but usually the top speed of 600 rpm does not allow a smooth surface to be produccd (and terrifies the patient!).

There are a variety of dental motors on the market, ranging from simple straight handpieces suitable for denture or orthodontic appliance trimming, to motors with foot switches suitable for prophylaxis. Portable conservation units, with micromotor, airotor and triple syringe, are available from several manufacturers, including a complete range by ADEC. Again, price is probably the limiting factor. The Eddystone unit is particularly straightforward and robust. It does, however, require to be powered by a small compressor or bottled compressed air. Its built-in suction is of the saliva-ejector type, but it can be used as a back-up unit in a surgery. In fact it is frequently supplied as the main dental unit in mobile surgeries.

Materials

Prosthetics

Alginate can be used just as easily in the home as in the surgery. Moist napkins and press-seal polythene bags will prevent distortion of impressions for some hours. For secondary impressions, the twin-tube, auto-mixing silicone impression materials are invaluable. There is no mixing or mess, and little need for cleaning the patient afterwards.

Soreness of the mucosa from an old denture can often be dealt with by easing the offending part and applying a tissue-conditioner, such as Viscogel, to the denture for the period between primary and secondary impression visits. This should also improve the quality of the impression.

Temporary chairside relines of self-cure acrylic, such as Total, are useful. Many uses for this material can be found (for example making post-dams; replacing fractured flanges) – enough to make it another permanent member of the prosthetics kit.

Conservation

It is possible to take an amalgamator on home visits, especially if it is the capsule-vibrating type; but the development of glass–ionomers and posterior composites means that most restorations can now be carried out in the home using only a selection of glass–ionomers or resins and a light-curing gun. The so-called compomers seem almost to have been developed specifically for domiciliary care. Metal-reinforced glass–ionomers such as Ketac Silver are often the restorative materials of choice for posterior occlusal and some two-surface restorations. The types of cavity most commonly found in elderly dentate people are cervical or root-face types, and these are most satisfactorily restored by adhesive glass–ionomers.

The development of command-set materials using the light-gun is a boon for home visits, and the whole restorative process can now take place without any mixing, waste or mess.

Useful accessories

Chair

Most homebound patients can be satisfactorily treated in their own chairs, but occasionally, when carrying out a large restoration, nothing is suitable. It is possible to use a portable chair, such as a garden recliner, but it must be capable of tilting the patient safely back to allow treatment from behind. It is also possible to use a camp-bed in a similar way. Bear in mind that if the patient is reclined, the dentist must also be seated low, and a folding fishing-stool can be ideal for this. It is also possible to sit on the equipment box if all else fails.

Safety equipment

There is just as much possibility of an emergency during dental care in a patient's home as in the surgery. An emergency kit should be carried, even if it is left in the car boot and not brought into the home each time. It is wise to keep adrenaline and hydrocortisone, plus suitable syringes and needles, in the equipment box permanently. A good case can be made for carrying oxygen in a small bottle (as designed for use by patients with respiratory problems), but this must be cleared with the insurance company for the vehicle in which it is to be carried.

It is sensible to take a fire extinguisher, of the type carried in cars, into the home if any form of naked flame is to be used for prosthetics. Sense has to be exercised. A safety-box or fire extinguisher left in the boot of a car parked outside the window is very much more convenient than one in a car parked in front of a city tower block 10 floors down.

Props and aids

Certain props and aids can be of use. One of the simplest is a 'thimble' made out of acrylic resin to protect the index finger of the non-working hand. This is made by heavily greasing (with Vaseline) the index finger and then moulding acrylic dough around it to make a thin but strong protective sleeve. If the finger is removed as the resin starts to heat up, the thimble can then be placed in hot water to set and then trimmed. A hole in the distal end threaded with string will secure it. The thimble can be used as a mouth-prop for patients unable to keep their mouths open, leaving the rest of the hand free to hold a mirror. This system is more flexible than using a conventional mouth-prop.

Cushions, pillows and bean-bags are used to prop patients up and keep them comfortable for half-an-hour or so. Headrests can be bought that clip over the arms of wheelchairs. However, a simple headrest can be made by attaching a car-seat head-restraint to a flat board. Strips of wood are attached with holes drilled in of a suitable size to take the supporting rods of the head-restraint. The board is then placed behind the patient, whose body weight holds it in place.

Yellow, strong polythene waste bags should always be taken to receive all waste sundries and materials. Leaving waste in the patient's home is unacceptable. Similarly, a small used-needle container must be carried. There are small square ones on the market. Polythene sandwich boxes with self-sealing lids are excellent for keeping syringes, napkins, cotton rolls, impression trays and all manner of small items that could otherwise be mislaid.

Clinical care

Palliative care

Pain-relief

The dentist's first priority should be to relieve pain. Pain is often the factor that causes the patient to request dental treatment in the first place, and adequate provision for it should be carried on the first visit. Carious cavities must be dressed with a sedative dressing such as zinc oxide/eugenol. Steroid-containing dressings such as Ledermix bring effective pain-relief, but their use should be confined to teeth to be extracted, as pulp death frequently follows their use.

Elderly patients usually have narrow root canals, and if a tooth becomes non-vital the usual characteristic sign (darkening of the dentine) may not be apparent, as so much secondary dentine is present. It can then often be difficult to identify the tooth responsible if the pain is not localized or there are no other features such as tenderness or mobility. This is a particular problem with lower incisors. An electric pulp-tester can be a good way of identifying non-vital teeth.

If the patient has an acute infection, the practice of opening up the pulp chamber to allow drainage may be impossible, and if a swelling is not amenable to incision, it may be necessary to resort to antibiotics until a handpiece and burs are available. Extraction of the tooth, particularly if it is loose, is much the best way to establish drainage.

If the pain is of denture origin, easing of the fitting surface is carried out. Pain-relief will also be rapid if the denture is left out until the ulcer or sore spot has healed, provided the cause of the ulcer has first been removed. Warm salt-water rinses are still the most useful agents to clear up traumatic soft tissue lesions. Agents, such as Difflam, with an anti-inflammatory action can have a place. Tissue conditioners such as Viscogel will rapidly ease the soreness caused by ill-fitting dentures, and their use for the homebound is recommended. It is important to follow up all denture-induced ulcers to make sure that they are healing as expected.

Treatment limitations

It is much easier to follow the rule of 'treat the patient and not the tooth' during home visits. Operative procedures require much planning and equipment, and questioning the need for each item of treatment should be automatic. Treatment plans should be based on the establishment of a working dentition that is easy for the patient to maintain. There is no need to restore teeth at all costs, and the presence of ten functional opposing pairs of teeth is probably all that is required.

Symptomless retained roots should not be routinely removed in the elderly housebound patient. If adjacent teeth are being extracted and the roots are loose, then there is no harm in extracting them. Otherwise, roots should be left alone unless their removal is essential. Lack of radiographic support and the unknown morphology of the roots complicates their removal to the point where it may be ill-advised.

Denture replacement must also be treated conservatively. Although the patient's old dentures may appear to cause extreme overclosure, they will probably have been that way for many years. Increases in face height should be limited to a maximum of 2 mm in a homebound person, or else they will not be tolerated.

Patients will be encountered who have a short life expectancy. Replacing worn yet otherwise satisfactory dentures for very elderly patients will leave them worse off than if no treatment had been undertaken. They will very often be unable to tolerate the new denture, yet have lost the facility they had with the old. Relines and tissue conditioner applications must be used to overcome soreness until the mucosa has healed. Although tissue conditioners are said to have a life of only a few weeks, it is often surprising how long their effect can be in selected cases, especially if allied to some careful easing. If possible, relining or re-basing should be tried first before replacing the denture of a housebound patient with a copy or one of a new design.

Patients dying before new dentures are completed are an upsetting but common experience when dental care is provided in homes for the elderly. Elderly or confused patients can be unable to co-operate sufficiently for new dentures to be made, especially if they have been without them for some time. Dentures constructed at the request of a relative or carer, without the interest or co-operation of the patient, are doomed to failure. Do not make dentures against your better judgment. When the dentures subsequently fail, explaining that they were made against your advice is a poor excuse. It is also worth remembering that many patients, through years of habituation, can cope with some astonishing designs. Do not replace problem-free dentures (however bizarre they may seem) just because they are not of the favoured design. The rule of 'if it works, leave it alone' is a sound one in domiciliary care.

Preventive care

Oral hygiene

People with mobility problems often have reduced manual dexterity, either through infirmity or as part of a handicapping condition. Oral hygiene problems are especially acute if the patient is dentate, and special care should be devoted to establishing satisfactory cleanliness as well as providing dietary advice.

Chemical agents

Fluoridated mouth rinses and anti-plaque agents are beneficial for people with poor brushing ability. Pre-brushing rinses containing Triclosan can reduce gingival inflammation and may be recommended. For patients with established gingival problems, chlorhexidine solutions and gels form part of the treatment regime, and their use on a regular basis is advisable.

Mechanical agents

Most toothbrushes have handles too thin to be grasped easily by an infirm or elderly hand. Handles may be thickened by wrapping with a length of adhesive fabric strapping, or securing a piece of foam pipe-lagging round them with elastic bands. Alternatively, bicycle hand-grips or rubber balls pushed over the handles provide a handle large enough for the disabled to grip.

The electric toothbrush here comes into its own. The large handle and the lack of need for intricate manipulation make it ideal for people with limited hand movements. It can be used reasonably well by a patient's carer, as it only needs to be held against the teeth to work effectively. If chlorhexidine gel is used once or twice a week instead of toothpaste, it is possible to maintain satisfactorily the oral health of the most severely disabled patient.

Chemo-mechanical agents

Although dental irrigators are not popular in the UK, they can be useful for a disabled patient with gingival problems. Dilute chlorhexidine solution placed in the reservoir penetrates to the base of periodontal pockets. Carers, too, find them easy to use.

Instructions to carers

Instructions to carers of disabled people must be of two types, depending on whether they only care for one person, or whether they are employed to look after many. For the carer with one patient, it is possible to demonstrate cleaning techniques on a one-to-one basis, advising on individual problems and solutions. This may take some time, particularly if a previously active person who has suffered a severe stroke is being cared for by his or her spouse, whose own manual dexterity may not be good. It usually only needs to be done once.

Where the carer is one of several who work in a home for the elderly or a hospital ward, then a different regime will be required. Staff will work separate shifts, and there will be a regular turnover of carers. Several visits must be made over a period of time to ensure that new staff are aware of problems. This can be undertaken by the practice Hygienist or well-trained Dental Surgery Assistant. The cleaning and care of dentures must be given a high priority.

Conservation

Caries removal

This is the stage at which most problems arise. Prosthetics, simple periodontal treatment and the extraction of loose teeth can all be carried out without extra equipment, but the cutting of cavities or the removal of defective fillings cannot be achieved without a dental motor. It is possible to cut enamel or amalgam with a bur in a slow handpiece attached to a standard laboratory motor or a portable laboratory mini-motor, but it is not recommended. The vibration is usually unacceptable for the patient, and safety is compromised. Most Community Dental Services in the UK possess equipment for domiciliary conservation, which they are only too happy to lend to interested general dental practitioners. Modern units usually have a high-speed handpiece with a water spray, an air motor and a triple syringe, all powered by a mini-compressor. Some even have built-in suction of the saliva-ejector variety.

Gross caries

Gross caries removal, particularly from the cervical area of the tooth, can often be completed without use of a bur. The prevalence of lesions of this type must increase in future, as more elderly people keep their teeth into old age. Caries is removed using only sharp medium and large straight excavators. No attempt is made to remove enamel unless it is very undermined and fragile. Wide, shallow cavities without clearly defined gingival borders must be restored with adhesive materials, and the glass–ionomers are particularly indicated. Good moisture control, adequate cavity conditioning and thorough drying (if necessary using compressed air in an aerosol sold for dust removal) are essential. Contamination of these cavities by moisture is not a great problem – hyposalivation is often present, and has contributed to the development of the carious lesions in the first place.

Rampant caries

Rampant caries is a widespread, rapidly-developing condition involving many of the teeth. Gross decalcification of the teeth in the cervical region can develop very rapidly in patients with hyposalivation. Drug-induced hyposalivation is common in old age. Caries develops rapidly, which can be painful for the patient and demoralizing for the dentist. Patients often resort to sucking mints or boiled sweets to try to make their mouths taste better, with disastrous results. Dietary counselling, prescription of an artificial saliva, cavity dressing with zinc oxide/eugenol temporary fillings and the application of fluoride varnishes to the remaining teeth are necessary to halt the rampant decay.

Moisture control

Moisture control in posterior cavities can be more of a problem on domiciliary visits than in the surgery, because of the absence of a high-velocity suction apparatus. Portable suction units are available, as used on hospital wards and for home nursing, but they are better suited to removing pools of liquid than saliva. A rubber dam can be invaluable on a home visit for isolating a tooth. Adhesive techniques and composite resins are very moisture-sensitive, and often a rubber dam is the only satisfactory solution. A couple of minutes applying the dam while the local anaesthetic is taking effect can save a strained temper and heroics with a fistful of cotton rolls during treatment. If a rubber dam is not used, Dry-guards may be of use.

Most types of restoration can be placed on domiciliary visits, including simple inlays, crowns and adhesive bridges. Whether they are ever appropriate is questionable. Use the ‘three year’ rule: i.e., if there is any suspicion that the restoration will need to be replaced within three years, it is better not to place it in the first instance. An alternative, such as extraction, should be considered. This is particularly true of cavities involving three or more surfaces, or those where the gingival floor is deep approximally. Working conditions in the home can never be as good as in the surgery, and the failed restoration often leads to a loss of confidence on both sides. It is better to aim for a simple maintainable dentition for the housebound patient, with the emphasis on function, than to try to preserve teeth at any cost.

Root canal therapy without radiographs is not recommended at any time. If essential, it may be possible to arrange for the patient to attend the surgery, and this is probably the only way in which endodontics should be carried out for the home-bound patient.

General attitude and patient–operator relationship

Adapting dental techniques refined in the controlled environment of the surgery to the variable and occasionally bizarre working place of a patient’s home can be very frustrating. Flexibility and patience beyond that usually required for dentistry are essential. The practitioner who likes a change from routine and is happy to improvise will almost certainly enjoy domiciliary treatment. The practitioner who becomes frustrated and irritated by equipment not performing as expected, and certain instruments not being available, will almost certainly loathe the vagaries of home visits. Spare instruments and alternatives can help to ease the occasional problem of dropping a vital instrument. A fixed routine of checking the contents of spirit lamps, cement bottles, impression materials and other consumables must be automatic.

A calm, unhurried style of treatment will greatly ease the patient and lighten the atmosphere. When home visits are booked at the end of a session, so that there is no time-pressure involved, this attitude can be maintained. The same clinical routine used with handicapped patients (tell, show, do), applies to the elderly and the infirm. Time taken to establish trust and rapport will be repaid over and over again in terms of the co-operation and relaxation of the patient.

Time spent at the initial vist in assessing the patient, the site and the working possibilities is also vital. The key to restorative domiciliary success is usually the ability to minimize the differences between home and surgery, and to optimize the patient's treatment position. Treatment planning should take these factors into account. Cushions, pillows and bean-bags should be used to prop the patient in a safe position, and their use should be noted in the patient record in order to speed up subsequent visits. Do not be shy of asking the patient to assume a position comfortable for you. Patients are grateful for home care, and usually understand that it is more difficult for the operator than the equivalent procedure in the surgery. The comfort of the operator can often be the limiting factor. Quality of treatment must suffer the more the operator is concerned with relieving his or her own pain rather than that of the patient.

Prosthetics

Preparation

Usually, for domiciliary care it is necessary to make a preliminary visit to examine the patient, take a full history, plan the treatment, and note any potential problems such as access, powerpoints, and visit times. Prosthetics is usually the one aspect of care where a start can also be made on the treatment, especially as the need for care is usually established at the first contact with the patient and his or her family or carer. Impression materials, trays, etc., and if possible a dental engine of some sort with acrylic trimmers should be taken, along with the standard mirror, probe and tweezers, plus a light-source.

Techniques

Every domiciliary visit carries a time and distance penalty for the dentist, so any procedure that can eliminate a visit is essential. However, far from its being a good idea to omit a visit for second impressions, this step is essential for domiciliary success. Only by the use of a close-fitting muscle-trimmed acrylic special tray with zinc oxide/eugenol or silicone wash can the usually resorbed ridges found in elderly housebound persons be recorded adequately. The fit of that denture will only be as good as the quality of the final impression, and time and effort spent at this stage will be repaid later. The omission of the second impression stage will almost certainly invite failure in domiciliary care, except in the hands of the most skilled practitioner. Eases carried out after the fitting of the denture are costly in terms of the time involved.

If existing dentures are reasonable, but have a worn occlusal surface – as often happens with dentures that have been in use for many years – a copy or replica technique is the treatment of choice. The main requirement for this is a dental technician familiar with the technique, plus soap dishes or oversized box impression trays suitable for taking an impression of the existing dentures. All the strictures of limiting face height increases to about 2 mm apply, even if the previous dentures were considerably overclosed. This is especially the case with the housebound patient, whose ability to cope with change may be limited by problems elsewhere in the body.

Usually, the majority of housebound patients can be treated in this way; but problems can occur with confused elderly patients who have mislaid their dentures altogether, particularly if they are ill-fitting and cause pain. This problem is more commonly found in residents of homes for the elderly or long-stay hospitals than in those in their own homes. The full prosthetic routine, as though for first-time dentures, is required, and it is vital that treatment commences as soon as possible. A confused elderly person who has successfully coped with full dentures for decades can lose this ability after only a few weeks. The prognosis for a new set is greatly worsened by delay.

Denture marking

The problem of lost dentures is an expensive and wasteful one that can be minimized with care. It is not uncommon for elderly patients to take their dentures out (especially the lower set) after lunch and lose them down the side of the chair. A simple denture-marking kit such as Gerident can save much time and repay its cost many times over by preventing mix-ups. Burring the gloss off a small part of the palate or lingual sulcus, writing the patient's initials with a soft pencil, and then covering with two coats of clear nail-varnish will identify a denture for some months, and is a cheap alternative. Better is to cut a channel, write the patient's name on the base, and cover it with autopolymerizing resin. Best of all is to incorporate the patient's name on a piece of tape (metal, plastic or even paper) within the denture at the flasking stage, so marking it for life.

Periodontics

Operative techniques

Scaling and root-planing are straightforward at home visits. If backed up with a simple dental engine, prolonged and satisfactory periodontal care (which will certainly be needed for homebound disabled people) can be undertaken with ease. A Cavitron ultrasonic scaler can be taken on domiciliary visits if it is fitted with a pressurized water vessel such as an adapted garden spray-gun. Reasonably efficient suction will be required.

Elderly and some disabled younger people who have retained any teeth will probably suffer tooth mobility to some degree. The level of mobility, the degree to which it causes problems, and the age of the patient must be considered. Careful scaling and root-planing will restore some firmness to mobile teeth in the absence of occlusal interference, but probably not for long; and this should be considered before subjecting the patient to the treatment.

Loose teeth should be extracted if they are causing pain or sepsis, and attention should be paid to the saveable ones. Again, aesthetics takes second place to function. Whilst molar teeth may be retained in the motivated healthy patient, even if there is bifurcation involvement, it is extremely unlikely that the homebound patient could maintain the oral hygiene necessary for long-term success.

Oral hygiene techniques

Adequate brushing is essential for periodontal therapy, and must be taken seriously. Carers may have to be taught how to do it for patients, standing or sitting behind them and using a mirror to check progress. It is far easier to brush another's teeth in the same way as one's own than trying to carry it out from in front.

Chlorhexidine gel has dramatically improved the prognosis for periodontally involved teeth in the homebound, and should be used regularly once or twice a week. If adequate brushing is not possible for a time – perhaps in the immediate aftermath of a stroke – then chlorhexidine gel can be rubbed in from the buccal side with a cotton roll or even a handkerchief.

Conclusions

The methods and equipment advocated above are not intended as a comprehensive solution for all possible situations. No mention has been made of mobile surgeries, specially equipped vans, portable X-ray units and other items unlikely to be possessed by the general practitioner. The vast majority of dentists are individualists, with the ability to adapt and create. Domiciliary dentistry gives the stimulus to do both. For the practitioner who may feel stifled by seeing the same four walls each day, an answer is to get beyond them and see patients in their own settings. To observe the lives others live is an education which is supplemented by the pleasure that comes from providing a high-quality service. In this way interest and pride in one's profession is maintained.

Bibliography

Andreason, J. O. and Andreason, F. M. (1990). *Essentials of Traumatic Injuries to the Teeth.* Munksgaard, Copenhagen.

Barbenel, J. C. (1974). The mechanics of the temporomandibular joint – a theoretical and electromyographic study. *J. Oral Rehabil.*, **1**, 19–27.

Berry, D. C. (1969). Mandibular dysfunction and chronic minor illness. *Br. Dent. J.*, **127**, 170–5.

Bessette, R. W., Bishop, B. and Mohl, N. (1973). Duration of the masseteric silent period in patient with temporomandibular joint syndrome. *J. Appl. Physiol.*, **30**, 864–9.

Bishop, M. (1993). Diagnostic imaging. In *Pathways in Practice*, pp. 11–24, Faculty of General Dental Practitioners, London.

Bullen, J. (1993). Records, negligence, consent and employment. In *Pathways in Practice*, pp. 137–144, Faculty of General Dental Practitioners, London.

Cox, P. J. and Rothwell, P. S. (1983). The masseteric silent period in subjects wearing acrylic bite plane. *J. Oral Rehabil.*, **10**, 51–5.

Cox, P. J., Rothwell, P. S. and Al-Khateeb, T. L. (1982). Measurement of masseteric silent periods after experimental bruxism. *J. Oral Rehabil.*, **5**, 487–92.

deBurgh Norman, J. E. and Bramley, P. A. (eds) (1990). *A Textbook and Colour Atlas of the Temporomandibular Joint. Diseases-Disorders-Surgery.* Wolfe Medical Publications, London.

Feinmann, C. and Harris, M. (1984). Psychogenic facial pain. *Br. Dent. J.*, **156**, 165–8, 205–8.

Fine, E. W. (1971). Psychological factors associated with non-organic temporomandibular pain dysfunction syndrome. *Br. Dent. J.*, **131**, 402–7.

Harkins, S. J. and Martenay, J. L. (1985). Extrinsic trauma: a significant factor in TMJ dysfunction. *J. Prosthet. Dent.*, **54**, 271–2.

Juniper, R. P. (1981). The superior pterygoid muscle? *Br. J. Oral Surg.*, **19**, 121–5.

Juniper, R. P. (1984). Temporomandibular joint dysfunction: a theory based upon electromyographic studies of the lateral pterygoid muscle. *Br. J. Oral Maxillofac. Surg.*, **22**, 1–8.

Kircof, L. T. (1987). Magnetic resonance imaging of the temporomandibular joint disc in asymptomatic volunteers. *J. Oral Maxillofac. Surg.*, **47**, 397–401.

Lamey, P. J. and Lewis, M. A. O. (1989). Oral medicine in practice: burning mouth syndrome. *Br. Dent. J.*, **167**, 197–200.

Lascelles, R. G. (1966). Atypical facial pain and depression. *Br. J. Psychiat.*, **112**, 651–9.

McGowan, D. A. (1990). Editorial. *Br. Dent. J.*, **169**, 3–4.

O'Brien, M. (1995). *Children's Dental Health in the United Kingdom 1993.* HMSO, London.

Ogus, H. (1975). Rheumatoid arthritis of the temporomandibular joint. *Br. J. Oral Surg.*, **12**, 275–84.

Poswillo Report (1990). *General Anaesthesia, Sedation and Resuscitation in Dentistry, Report of an Expert Working Party.*

Redfield, R. R., Wright, D. C. and Tramont, E. C. (1986). The Walter Reed staging classification for HTLV-111/LAV infection. *New Engl. J. Med.*, **341**, 131–2.

Rees, L. A. (1954). The structure and function of the mandibular joint. *Br. Dent. J.*, **96**, 125–33.

Rothwell, P. S. (1980). DDS Thesis, Manchester University.

Rothwell, P. S. (1987). Symptoms of pain dysfunction in 400 patients; time to revise the classical profile? *J. Dent.*, **15**, 6–11.

Toller, P. A. (1973). Osteoarthrosis of the mandibular condyle. *Br. Dent. J.*, **134**, 223–31.

Index